SPEECH AND LANGUAGE DISORDERS

COMMUNICATION SKILLS

CHALLENGES, IMPORTANCE FOR HEALTH CARE PROFESSIONALS AND STRATEGIES FOR IMPROVEMENT

SPEECH AND LANGUAGE DISORDERS

Additional books in this series can be found on Nova's website under the Series tab.

Additional e-books in this series can be found on Nova's website under the e-books tab.

SPEECH AND LANGUAGE DISORDERS

COMMUNICATION SKILLS

CHALLENGES, IMPORTANCE FOR HEALTH CARE PROFESSIONALS AND STRATEGIES FOR IMPROVEMENT

BRIDGET L. WRIGHT
EDITOR

NOVA BIOMEDICAL

New York

Library of Congress Cataloging-in-Publication Data

Names: Wright, Bridget L., editor.
Title: Communication skills : challenges, importance for health care professionals and strategies for improvement / editor, Bridget L. Wright.
Description: Hauppauge, New York : Nova Science Publisher's, Inc., [2016] | Series: Speech and language disorders | Includes bibliographical references and index.
Identifiers: LCCN 2016024901 (print) | LCCN 2016028619 (ebook) | ISBN 9781634855655 (softcover) | ISBN 9781634855792 (ebook) | ISBN 9781634855792 ()
Subjects: LCSH: Communication in medicine. | Interpersonal communication. | Language disorders. | Physician and patient.
Classification: LCC R118 .C6184 2016 (print) | LCC R118 (ebook) | DDC 610--dc23
LC record available at https://lccn.loc.gov/2016024901

Published by Nova Science Publishers, Inc. † New York

CONTENTS

PREFACE

The authors of this book provide current research on the challenges of communication skills, its importance for health care professionals and strategies for improvement. Chapter One explores the literature that studies the impact of electronic medical record use on communication between physicians and patients. Chapter Two reviews communicating with the psychologically distressed patient. Chapter Three reviews major theories of neurocommunication intended as the application of the findings of neurosciences for the study of interprofessional communication and behavior in healthcare. Chapter Four studies decision-making models in patients with depression.

Chapter 1 – There has been tremendous increase in the use of electronic medical record (EMR) in the past decade. Despite its wide implementation and potential benefits on cost and quality of care, there still exists debate on the impact of electronic record use and physician patient communication. In this chapter, the authors will explore the literature that studies the impact of electronic medical record use on communication between the physician and patient. There is no doubt that the introduction of the computer into the physician's office has introduced a third party in the interview and this required new set of communication skills that needs to be learned. This chapter will describe the needed skills that take into consideration the new triad of doctor-patient-computer: coordination between gaze at the screen and eye contact with the patient; maintain balance between attending to the patient and using the computer, room configuration for better sharing of the computer screen and distraction of the physician by typing and reading the electronic chart.

Chapter 2 – Mental health problems are prevalent in primary care; yet they are under-recognized. This leads to significant morbidity and higher services utilization. Effective communication skills (CS) are of paramount importance to detect psychological distress and achieve better patient adherence to medications and health outcomes. Specific CS that aid in detecting and dealing with psychologically distressed patients in the primary care setting are highlighted. Legitimizing concerns, allowing for silence, adopting a patient centered biopsychosocial model, and addressing emotions, are important skills when attending to patients with mental diseases. A review of the BATHE technique is given as one way to ensure that primary care physicians address psychosocial issues. The use of the acronym N-U-R-S-E helps health professionals address emotions appropriately. A visual aid that may help patients understand the link between the body and mind and improve adherence to treatment is described.

Chapter 3 – Recent developments in the neurosciences are offering an exclusive revision of all social and humanistic sciences. These also include psychology, counseling, mental health, and communication sciences. The idea that specific areas within the brain are activated during social interactions and communication is not recent. However, the brain has been found to record, react, and respond in unique and measurable ways when two or more people cooperate. In addition, prosocial behaviors, interpersonal communication, and teamwork also respond to a complex neurointegration of signals generated by the pairing of participants' brains, environment, and behavior. This chapter summarizes the major contributions that the neural sciences can provide to the understanding and improvement of prosocial communication and collaboration in healthcare and interprofessional teamwork. Prosocial communication for healthcare providers can be demanding and challenging. In fact, the participants in interprofessional activities should share proper communication skills to allow profitable interactions. Furthermore, they are also asked to integrate their behavior, attitudes, and expectations in order to promote the same communication milieu in the group. The neural mechanisms endorsing these adaptations are complex. However, recent advancements in the neurosciences allow an understanding of how the human brain functions in prosocial communication. Additionally, it is possible to stimulate group behavior that activates specific areas within the brain. This chapter will review major theories of neurocommunication intended as the application of the findings of neurosciences for the study of interprofessional communication and behavior in healthcare. All cerebral areas will be reconsidered in greater detail regarding their contribution to prosocial communication. Further details will be provided about instruments to study team interactions by recording group EEG or hyperscanning and neurocardiac studies on Heart Rate Variability (HRV) and Peripheral Oxygenation Variability (POV) during prosocial communication. In this chapter, the authors define communication neuroscience in interprofessional teamwork as the study of brain activities that determine prosocial communication, behaviors, skills, attitudes, and emotions of healthcare professionals involved in a collaborative practice. In this respect, the contribution of all cerebral areas is reconsidered as well as their influences on behaviors during interactive communication. This neurocommunicational perspective adds insight into the brain's functions that influence therapeutic and professional speech and listening. From here, neuroeducation can start with the intent to pair specific communication behaviors with the corresponding cerebral areas. The gain is a holistic and neurobehavioral theory of communication. The advantage is an understanding of that objective and neuroanatomical basis that generates and improves communication. The challenge is the creation of Neurocommunication Labs that allow the development of prosocial communication by understanding and training the social brain.

Chapter 4 – The clinical decision process is central to the patient-physician relationship. The paternalistic approach, once the preferential model of medical practice is now under severe criticism. Clinicians find themselves trying to find alternative models where the physician is not a sole source of information as in an Informed Decision Model, nor an agent to interpret the will and decide by the patient as in a Doctor-as-Agent Model. The Shared-Decision Model is in line with this endeavor, inviting the patient and physician to be co-responsible with the information exchange and treatment plan.

This model, based on strong communication ability, shows particular interest in the decisions that are sensitive to personal preferences and entail some degree of uncertainty – as the majority of the decisions made in the psychiatric field. Furthermore depression is thought to place patient's capability to decide at risk. The research shows however that patients with depression still want to participate in the clinical decisions, and reports a positive impact of using this model on the compliance with the therapeutic plan, in a decreased need of hospitalization and in better knowledge of the illness and higher satisfaction with health services. Shared-decision appears to be of additional interest, once it promotes the sense of autonomy and self-efficacy, decreasing feelings of helplessness and hopelessness associated with depressive state.

The authors performed a review of the models of decision making and its application to psychiatric patients. The reviewed literature permited to uncover the model characteristics more suitable to application in depressed patients and their physicians in the decision process. When dealing with patients with depression, sharing technical knowledge and information and the joined participation in the process of decision seems to be welcomed, and even desired. Results highlight the influence of a Shared-Decision Model on patient's satisfaction and compliance with treatment.

In: Communication Skills
Editor: Bridget L. Wright

ISBN: 978-1-63485-565-5

Chapter 1

COMMUNICATION SKILLS IN THE ERA OF THE ELECTRONIC MEDICAL RECORDS: CHALLENGES AND OPPORTUNITIES

Jumana Antoun[1,*], MD, MS, and Jad Aridi[2,†], MD

[1]Department of Family Medicine, American Univesrity of Beirut, Beirut,Lebanon

[2]Physician, Beirut, Lebanon

ABSTRACT

There has been tremendous increase in the use of electronic medical record (EMR) in the past decade. Despite its wide implementation and potential benefits on cost and quality of care, there still exists debate on the impact of electronic record use and physician patient communication. In this chapter, we will explore the literature that studies the impact of electronic medical record use on communication between the physician and patient. There is no doubt that the introduction of the computer into the physician's office has introduced a third party in the interview and this required new set of communication skills that needs to be learned. This chapter will describe the needed skills that take into consideration the new triad of doctor-patient-computer: coordination between gaze at the screen and eye contact with the patient; maintain balance between

* Corresponding author: Address: Department of Family Medicine, American University of Beirut, PO BOX 110236, Beirut, Lebanon. Email ja46@aub.edu.lb.

† Address: Beirut, Lebanon. Email jad.aridi1@gmail.com.

attending to the patient and using the computer, room configuration for better sharing of the computer screen and distraction of the physician by typing and reading the electronic chart.

Keywords: communication skills, electronic medical record, training

1. INTRODUCTION

1.1. Importance of Communication Skills

Few would argue against the importance of the physician–patient relationship when it comes to providing successful, durable, high-quality health care. This concept is not only intuitive, but has also been supported by data from many studies [1-4]. Patients who report good physician communication provide more detailed histories, follow their physician's advice, and adhere better with the treatment regimen [2]. Not only does a good relationship between patients and their physician lead to a better clinical outcome especially when dealing with chronic illnesses, it also results in higher satisfaction for the physician, less stress on the job and lower rates of malpractice lawsuits from the patients [2]. In an effort to optimize this relationship for maximal efficiency, the American Academy on Physician and Patient held a conference in 2002 in Kalamzoo, Michigan. This conference produced a consensus on a set of communication and interpersonal skills required to conduct a successful medical interview and establish a high functioning patient–physician relationship [5]. However, a new variable has been added to an adaptable equation and that is the rise of the electronic medical records (EMR).

1.2. Patient-Physician-Computer Triad

The rise of heavy computerization in almost all fields of work did not spare the medical community. Computers emerged as a powerful tool to manage, organize and archive patient records, and later developed into Health Information Technologies, with Electronic Medical Records (EMR) being a major component of these technologies [6]. Soon, most physicians started adopting the EMR in their clinic. This resulted in a shift of the nature of the relationship with the patient from a dyadic communication into a triad. Every corner of this triad contributes to the outcome of the medical interview, and the interaction between the three components influences the encounter [7].

Although physicians have their concerns about the impact of the computer on the patient-doctor relationship, most of these concerns were dissipated after the implementation of the electronic medical records [8]. Interestingly, physicians change their regular behaviors to overcome the possible impediments to communication posed by the presence of the computer [8]. Analysis of videotaped encounters showed that physicians tend to move between a dyadic relationship when discussing intimate subjects with patients to a more triadic relationship when discussing prescription of laboratory results [9]. Furthermore, Frankel et al. showed that the EMR use did not affect physician-patient communication but rather amplified the baseline communication skills whether negative or positive [10]. Physicians who had good baseline skills were able to continue to give attention to their patients even after the introduction of the computer.

In view of these complex interactions, that seem to be deeply affecting the classical medical interview conduction, and given the importance of this encounter on the outcomes of patient care, it is important to review the benefits and risks of EMR use in the clinic and contemplate the possible interventions that could increase the benefits.

2. Negative Effects of EMR on Communication

2.1. Patient Centeredness

The design of the medical interview culminated in the concept of patient centeredness where the patient is incorporated into that process as an active member, especially in the areas of decision-making and therapeutic course modeling [11] which was found to yield higher success in terms of care delivery. The introduction of the EMR showed detrimental effects on the patient centeredness of that exchange, resulting in the physician losing rapport with the patient [12]. The introduction of the EMR has, therefore, been associated with an increase in the number and complexity of tasks required from the physician during the interview. These complex tasks intruded on the delicate nature of the physician-patient relationship due to the difficulty of multitasking and dividing his/her attention between the computer and patient [13].

Furthermore, physicians tended to use the EMR as a way to avoid addressing the psychosocial aspect or the illness's effect on the patient's life [13]. The patient might divulge personal, emotional or psychological problems, and these should be addressed. Research has found, however, that these issues are not as well spoken to in the presence of the computer [14]. It is recommended that the undivided attention should be focused on the patient when such matters are being explored, with hands off the mouse and keyboard and eyes off the screen with no reference to the computer [15].

2.2. The Interview's Opening Minute

It has been noted that the disruption to the patient – physician interaction in the presence of the computer starts at the very beginning of the interview process, within the first minute. The beginning of the interview, which sets the tone, became a composite of three players: the physician, the patient and the computer, all three interacting [16]. It has also been shown that many physicians walked straight to their computer upon entering the consultation room using it as their opening statement instead of inciting the patient to share their story and concern [17]. That again could have negative ramifications on the interaction between the physician and the patient as well as the flow of the rest of the interview. It is, therefore, helpful to acknowledge the patient before reverting to the computer by extending a friendly greeting upon entering, introducing the computer into the encounter, and reassuring the patient of its confidentiality when necessary.

2.3. Eye Contact, Screen Gaze and Non-Verbal Cues

A major determinant in establishing a relationship between patient and physician is non-verbal communication with eye contact being an important aspect. The presence of the computer in the consultation room has had a noticeable and important impact on that area of the medical encounter [18]. Screen gazing while talking or listening to the patient was inversely proportional to the depth of exploring the patient's emotional issues, view of their medical problem, and setting up an agenda for the encounter [12]. Screen gazing was found to take 25-40% of the interview in some cases [14] and was negatively correlated with patient centeredness of the interview. Screen gazing was found to negatively affect the interaction with the patient by reducing the doctor's emotional involvement in the interview process and thereby affecting its outcome.

It is, therefore, clear that physicians should be conscious and wary about their screen gazing throughout the interview and make sure to alternate their focus between the patient and the screen. This behavior assures the patient that they are being actively listened to and their troubles and worries are not being dismissed which strengthens the non-verbal bond. Moreover, physicians should optimize their operational computer skills so that they can smoothly alternate between the computer and the patient without being worried about technical difficulties.

Empathy is another major component of the set of interpersonal skills. It has been shown to be a significant booster of adherence and positive outcomes [17]. Since EMR has been shown to negatively affect these sentiments, [14] special care should be taken not to lose track of the ultimately caring and genuinely compassionate nature of the physician's approach. Non-verbal clues should also be incorporated in the interaction to indicate active listening and understanding of the patient's problems. Signals can be used to maintain contact with the patient while using the computer such as alternation of gaze, nodding, and verbal signals of shifting to the computer without diverting one's attention to the patient's needs [17]. All of these can be maintained while typing on the computer to remain efficient and attentive to the patient's needs

2.4. Spatial Configuration

Just as the impact of non-verbal communication can be significant on the physician-patient relationship, the consultation room's spatial organization may also affect it. It may serve as a facilitator or an obstruction in the face of the free-flowing dialogue between the patient and the doctor. When a third party is added, optimizing the spatialconfiguration of the room becomes paramount so that the physician, the patient and the computer would have a straightforward communication pathway [16]. Not only would the organization of the room have a direct effect on the unfolding of the interview, but it would also affect eye contact and sharing of information indirectly. The position of the computer within the room has revealed many challenges. First, when the EMR is accessible to the physician, he/she showed a tendency to input the data provided immediately and to pay less attention to the patient. Second, the location of the computer might result in obstructed eye contact and, sometimes, may impede the ability of the physician to face the patient, forcing both the physicians and patients to move their chairs or lean their bodies which caused significant breaks in the conversation [12]. A welcoming and open spatial configuration to the room with the patient able to view the information on the screen would promote a successful start to the physician-patient encounter [12, 16, 17].

3. Advantages of the EMR in the Medical Interview

EMRs have been shown to improve the quality of care in some areas, especially in care coordination among care–givers and cost reduction mainly by decreasing errors of miscommunication [19]. It also helps in increasing accuracy and clarity of prescription orders [20]. The benefits that are of higher importance are the ones within the confines of the medical interview, and that specifically affect the relationship between patient and physician.

3.1. Patient Engagement

Possibly one of the most important aspects of the medical consultation is the level of patient engagement in their treatment and their involvement in the patient-physician relationship. The ability of the patients to feel safe and comfortable to participate in their own care is not to be underestimated. A plan crafted by the patient and physician together, one whose pitfalls and risks they understand well, is a plan that the patients are more likely to adhere to and manage better. The use of the EMR in consultation has enhanced that aspect of the interview, especially when the physician is willing and able to share the information registered in the EMR and encourages the patient's interaction during the interview process [21].

Sharing the screen with the patient and pointing to relevant data as they are asked open-ended questions has been found to strengthen the forming relationship [22]. In the presence of EMR, there were more open-ended questions from the physician, increased use of the partnership approach, as well as an increase in positive and social talks. It has also helped the physician ensure the completion of his/her notes by sharing the screen and allowing the patient to amend or rectify any errors as well as add any missing information [21].

3.2. Sharing Information

The use of EMR has brought along an improvement in information exchange between patients and physicians in the form of encouraging questions, improved discussions about therapy, and patient counseling [12, 20, 23]. This behavior should be praised and reinforced for it helps to maximize the profitable use of the EMR, involves the patient in its management and strengthens the patient-physician relationship. EMR does provide a certain structure to stored information. When physicians are comfortable with EMR use and application, it proves to be a helpful tool in certain aspects of the medical interview. Physicians using EMR were found to be more active in delivering information about the patients' illnesses as well as sharing the patient's progress while following specific therapeutic regimens [18]. These physicians were also found to be more active in clarifying ambiguous concepts and encouraging patients to ask questions and be involved in the therapeutic regimen [10, 18]. Since establishing a partnership between a patient and physician is of paramount importance to the healthy functioning of the medical encounter, the introduction of the computer into the triadic relationship has positively affected information sharing and discussion between these two individuals.

It has also been shown that EMR has assisted in clearer discussions regarding medications, their indication, side effects, mode and frequency of administration, resulting in higher patient adherenceto the suggested regimen [24]. Screen sharing also allowed physicians to use tools such as risk calculators, graphs or other visual aids to help educate the patient about their illnesses, progress and management.

3.3. Familiarity and General Satisfaction

Among the studies undertaken on the subject of EMR influence on the physician-patient relationship, it has been found that patients' general satisfaction of their physician's use of EMR in the medical interview has improved. This is because the patients' understanding of the encounter all together increased with a higher level of assurance about dealing with their illnesses, especially the chronic ones. The familiarity of their physicians with their conditions, fueled by the information available to physicians through the EMR, also helped improve this general feeling of satisfaction with the unfolding of the interview [2].

It should be noted that it is important for the physician to understand the patient's perspective towards the computer in the consultation and to modulate its use and perhaps eliminate it completely if needed [9]. Some patients may be uncomfortable with its presence, which could lead to a partial collapse of the relationship with adverse or unsatisfying outcomes of the interview.

4. Electronic Health Records in Medical Training

With all this in mind, the impact of the computer in the medical interview as an active member of triad could easily enhance or impede the development and outcome of the encounter and have ramification on the patients' health and illness management. Given the importance of such a participant, it is vital to elucidate a few areas. How can a physician minimize the negative aspects and optimize the use of EMR within the setting of the medical interview?

EMRs, by themselves, would not directly provide either the benefits or the harm discussed above. It all depends on the end user. A physician who is not exposed to them or trained to use them appropriately is a physician more likely to get lost in the EMR and lose focus from the intended purpose of the medical interview [25]. The physician-patient interaction, in the presence of the computer, depends on the physician's baseline skills and the introduction of the computer only serves to amplify them. This theory specifically applies to the visit's organization as well as the physician's verbal and non-verbal behavior towards the patient. Physicians who were comfortable integrating note-taking and chart-filling while gathering information from the patient easily transitioned these skills in the presence of the computer. However, others who initially had trouble with combining these two aspects of the interview faced further trouble when the computer was introduced into the picture [10]. Another important factor to be considered is the physician's typing skills and ease of accessing information from an electronic database. These skills also proved to be important in facilitating the introduction of the EMR and its flow into the medical encounter [10, 26].

With the unavoidable rise in prevalence of EMR, it is crucial that physicians in training develop Health Information Technology competencies [27]. Not only are these competencies necessary to keep up with the demands of such systems technically, but it is also necessary to keep these technologies from becoming an obstacle in the relationship and management of the physician-patient encounter.

Table 1. Set of EMR specific communication skills required to be completed by health care professional during the medical interview process in the presence of the computer

Communication Skills
Setting the stage
Greet patient appropriately and acknowledge waiting time if needed
Illicit chief complaint before turning to the computer
Introduce the computer into the Doctor-Patient-Computer triad
Explain and reassure patient of confidentiality of EMR
Rearrange spatial configuration so computer does not obstruct communication (screen in comfortable sharing position, physician not turning back to the patient …)
Eliciting Information
Explore the patient's psychosocial background
Intermittently look at computer for previous relevant information while interviewing the patient
Point to relevant areas on the screen when needed
Avoid computer use when patient is addressing a concern with a significant psychological burden
Involve patient in verifying EMR data entry's accuracy and completion
Giving Information
When sharing the screen, physician should verify the patient's ability to visualize the contents optimally
Discuss patient's results with on-screen visual aids (graphs, charts …)
Encourage patient to ask questions and check for patient understanding
Share patient's educational material using electronic resources
Keep balanced eye contact within the triad while sharing information
Understand Patient's perspective
Recognize the patient's perspective on the use of the computer in the clinic and act accordingly
End Encounter
Provide handouts or website references and community support services, medication side effects, etc.

Integrating the use of EMR into medical training will allow graduating physicians to consider these complex information systems as part of their daily routine. This will make EMR a much easier tool to use and incorporate in the interview [28]. While these measures seem necessary to ensure a complete medical education, reports show that EMR are still very minimally integrated, if at all, in most medical education systems [27, 29].

5. Suggested Curricula for EMR Specific Communication Skills

Given the meteoric rise of EMR use in medical practice, its importance regarding the physician-patient relationship, and the potential pitfalls of its introduction to the medical encounter, it is important to ensure the proper handling of such a tool. With that purpose in mind, the introduction of a set of EMR specific communication skills is necessary to at least guarantee the conservation of a meaningful and fruitful physician-patient relationship where the computer is described as a third partner, useful in advancing and improving the outcome of such relationship, rather than hindering it. This set of skills is illustrated in Table 1. This set of skills has been guided by both the Kalamazoo report [5] and based on the SEGUE framework of setting the stage, eliciting information, giving information, understanding the patient's perspective and ending the encounter [26].

Conclusion

The computer has crashed into the intimate relationship that exists between a patient and physician. It certainly brings with it a host of advantages, but it also heralds a possible breakdown of this relationship if not managed properly. Physicians should utilize their communication and interpersonal skills to veer the presence of the computer in the medical interview away from its harmful capabilities and towards its benefits through its integration in the newborn triad. This could not be ensured without first introducing EMR use into medical curricula and training physicians on the most effective way of using them. The priority is to maintain a continuous patient-centered interview organized into a well-set stage for enhanced and comprehensive information gathering, appropriate use of the computer, and most importantly, a thorough understanding of the patient's perspective. In short, it is vital for the physician to remember his/her essential role as a care provider and conserve his/her sense of empathy instead of focusing on practicality and technology.

REFERENCES

[1] Committee on Quality of Health Care in American IoM. *Crossing the Quality Chasm: A New Health System for the 21st Century*. Washington, Dc: National Academy Press; 2001.

[2] Ha JF, Longnecker N. Doctor-patient communication: a review. *Ochsner J* 2010;10(1):38-43.

[3] Lansky D. Measuring what matters to the public. *Health Aff* (Millwood) 1998 Jul;17(4):40-1.

[4] Robbins JA, Bertakis KD, Helms LJ, Azari R, Callahan EJ, Creten DA. The influence of physician practice behaviors on patient satisfaction. *Fam Med* 1993 Jan;25(1):17-20.

[5] Duffy FD, Gordon GH, Whelan G, Cole-Kelly K, Frankel R, Buffone N, et al. Assessing competence in communication and interpersonal skills: the Kalamazoo II report. *Acad Med* 2004 Jun;79(6):495-507.

[6] Blumenthal D, Glaser JP. Information technology comes to medicine. *N Engl J Med* 2007 Jun 14;356(24):2527-34.

[7] Scott D, Purves IN. Triadic relationship between doctor, computer and patient. *Interacting with computers* 8[4], 347-363. 1996.

[8] Doyle RJ, Wang N, Anthony D, Borkan J, Shield RR, Goldman RE. Computers in the examination room and the electronic health record: physicians' perceived impact on clinical encounters before and after full installation and implementation. *Fam Pract* 2012 Oct;29(5):601-8.

[9] Pearce C, Arnold M, Phillips C, Trumble S, Dwan K. The patient and the computer in the primary care consultation. *J Am Med Inform Assoc* 2011 Mar;18(2):138-42.

[10] Frankel R, Altschuler A, George S, Kinsman J, Jimison H, Robertson NR, et al. Effects of exam-room computing on clinician-patient communication: a longitudinal qualitative study. *J Gen Intern Med* 2005 Aug;20(8):677-82.

[11] Pearce C, Dwan K, Arnold M, Phillips C, Trumble S. Doctor, patient and computer - a framework for the new consultation. *Int J Med Inform* 2009 Jan;78(1):32-8.

[12] Shachak A, Reis S. The impact of electronic medical records on patient-doctor communication during consultation: a narrative literature review. *J Eval Clin Pract* 2009 Aug;15(4):641-9.

[13] Booth N, Robinson P, Kohannejad J. Identification of high-quality consultation practice in primary care: the effects of computer use on doctor-patient rapport. *Inform Prim Care* 2004;12(2):75-83.

[14] Margalit RS, Roter D, Dunevant MA, Larson S, Reis S. Electronic medical record use and physician-patient communication: an observational study of Israeli primary care encounters. *Patient Educ Couns* 2006 Apr;61(1):134-41.

[15] Pearce C, Walker H, O'Shea C. A visual study of computers on doctors' desks. *Inform Prim Care* 2008;16(2):111-7.

[16] Pearce C, Trumble S, Arnold M, Dwan K, Phillips C. Computers in the new consultation: within the first minute. *Fam Pract* 2008 Jun;25(3): 202-8.

[17] Duke P, Frankel RM, Reis S. How to integrate the electronic health record and patient-centered communication into the medical visit: a skills-based approach. *Teach Learn Med* 2013;25(4):358-65.

[18] Silverman J, Kinnersley P. Doctors' non-verbal behaviour in consultations: look at the patient before you look at the computer. *Br J Gen Pract* 2010 Feb;60(571):76-8.

[19] Burton LC, Anderson GF, Kues IW. Using electronic health records to help coordinate care. *Milbank Q* 2004;82(3):457-81, Table.

[20] McGrath JM, Arar NH, Pugh JA. The influence of electronic medical record usage on nonverbal communication in the medical interview. *Health Informatics J* 2007 Jun;13(2):105-18.

[21] Crampton NH, Reis S, Shachak A. Computers in the clinical encounter: a scoping review and thematic analysis. *J Am Med Inform Assoc* 2016 Jan 14.

[22] Baker LH, O'connell D, Platt FW. "What else?" Setting the agenda for the clinical interview. *Ann Intern Med* 2005 Nov 15;143(10):766-70.

[23] Makoul G, Curry RH, Tang PC. The use of electronic medical records: communication patterns in outpatient encounters. *J Am Med Inform Assoc* 2001 Nov;8(6):610-5.

[24] Arar NH, Wen L, McGrath J, Steinbach R, Pugh JA. Communicating about medications during primary care outpatient visits: the role of electronic medical records. *Inform Prim Care* 2005;13(1):13-22.

[25] Barnett JS. Incorporating electronic medical records into the physician assistant educational curriculum. *J Physician Assist Educ* 2013;24(2): 48-54.

[26] Skillings JL, Porcerelli JH, Markova T. Contextualizing SEGUE: Evaluating Residents' Communication Skills Within the Framework of a Structured Medical Interview. *J Grad Med Educ* 2010 Mar;2(1):102-7.

[27] Graham-Jones P, Jain SH, Friedman CP, Marcotte L, Blumenthal D. The need to incorporate health information technology into physicians'

education and professional development. *Health Aff* (Millwood) 2012 Mar;31(3):481-7.

[28] Kushniruk AW, Borycki EM, Armstrong B, Joe R, Otto T. Bringing electronic patient records into health professional education: towards an integrative framework. *Stud Health Technol Inform* 2009;150:883-7.

[29] Kushniruk AW, Borycki EM, Armstrong B, Joe R, Otto T. Bringing electronic patient records into health professional education: towards an integrative framework. *Stud Health Technol Inform* 2009;150:883-7.

In: Communication Skills
Editor: Bridget L. Wright

ISBN: 978-1-63485-565-5

Chapter 2

COMMUNICATING WITH THE PSYCHOLOGICALLY DISTRESSED PATIENT

Basem Roberto Saab*[1], *MD*, and *Jumana Antoun*[2], *MD, MS

[1]Professor
[2]Assistant Professor
Department of Family Medicine,
American University of Beirut Medical Center, Beirut, Lebanon

ABSTRACT

Mental health problems are prevalent in primary care; yet they are under-recognized. This leads to significant morbidity and higher services utilization. Effective communication skills (CS) are of paramount importance to detect psychological distress and achieve better patient adherence to medications and health outcomes. Specific CS that aid in detecting and dealing with psychologically distressed patients in the primary care setting are highlighted. Legitimizing concerns, allowing for silence, adopting a patient centered biopsychosocial model, and addressing emotions, are important skills when attending to patients with mental diseases. A review of the BATHE technique is given as one way to ensure that primary care physicians address psychosocial issues. The use of the acronym N-U-R-S-E helps health professionals address emotions appropriately. A visual aid that may help patients understand the link between the body and mind and improve adherence to treatment is described.

1. INTRODUCTION

1.1. Mental Illness in Primary Care

Mental health problems are prevalent in primary care. Due to the stigma of consulting psychiatrists and the ill-defined symptoms of mental problems, patients tend to visit the primary care physician. Missing mental health problems in primary care is attributed to the fact that two-third of patients with depression have somatic symptoms. [1] Failure to diagnose patients with mental illness leads to significant morbidity and higher services utilization [2-4]. The US Preventive Services Task Force recommends depression screening of the general adult population on condition of the presence of adequate system to ensure accurate diagnosis and treatment. [5] There are several screening tools to detect mental health problem [6, 7].

1.2. Communication Skills and Mental Illness

Good communication skills (CS) are of paramount importance in health care delivery. Plato alluded to this as early as 300 BC. Plato described the free doctor as a person who will not prescribe a drug to his patient before convincing the patient and his companions of the value of treatment. [8] Interpersonal and communication skills is one of the six competencies that are stated by the Accreditation Council for Graduate Medical Education in the United States. [9] Effective CS has been shown to lead to better patient adherence to medication and patient reported outcomes [10-12].

In one focus group study, adult patients emphasized the importance of an empathic relationship with the provider and expressed their expectation of good CS from their physicians when choosing their provider for mental health. [13] Thus acquiring good CS is even more important when dealing with mental health patients. This chapter will highlight the importance of the use of some of the basic communication skills in the context of interviewing a psychologically distressed patient (PDP) at the primary care level. The skills will be grouped into functions rather than their chronological use during the encounter.

2. Communication Skills That Help to Detect Psychological Distress

2.1. Attention to Non-Verbal Clues

The ability to detect non-verbal clues increases the likelihood of detecting a mental health problem. [14] For example, an elderly man with a blunt face, unshaved beard brought by his daughter for weight loss to the clinic should alert the physician to the possibility of depression. Missing these clues to diagnose depression might end up with ordering several unnecessary tests. It is also as important that the physician pays attention to his/her own non-verbal responses and maintains a relaxed posture [15].

2.2. Biopsychosocial Approach

Addressing the psychosocial aspects without neglecting the biological aspects assures the patient that the physician is taking care of her/him as a person and not just another patient or customer. The physician can use the acronym N-U-R-S-E to address emotions. It stands for naming the effect/emotion, showing understanding and respect, as well as supporting and empathizing with the patient. Also, having a thorough psychosocial history can significantly sharpen the diagnosis and reduce health expenses [16].

> N-U-R-S-E approach while communicating with a 32-year-old patient who has an adjustment disorder with anxiety symptoms after her husband has lost his work.
>
> Patient: (talking rapidly and looks apprehensive) Could this chest pain be due a heart problem?
>
> Dr.: You seem worried and afraid. (Name the emotion). Are you afraid that this pain could be related to heart problem?
>
> Patient: Yes, I am afraid I am having a heart attack
>
> Dr.: Your point is well taken. (Respect her fear) Why do you think this could be related to heart problem? (Understand her fear)
>
> Patient: It is always advertised that chest pain may indicate a heart attack. I have a family to take care of.
>
> Dr.: Any mother passing through tough times, dealing with the laying off of her husband from work, would feel afraid and worried. (Empathize) You have now more responsibility to take care of the family.

Yet, I would like to reassure you that the possibility of heart attack is a remote possibility taking into consideration the quality, duration, pain location, and your age.

Patient: How can you explain this pain?

Dr.: [explaining the mind-body model…] I will teach you some breathing exercises to deal with the chest pain. I am always available if you need further help. We can always talk about what is bothering you and how to deal with the situation (Support).

BATHE technique is a simple technique devised by Stuart and Lieberman useful for patients with psychosocial problems. [17] BATHE stands for background, affect, trouble, handle and empathy. It is important to let the patient talk initially without interruption and to explore the physical complaint thoroughly before addressing the psychosocial background. For example, after questioning about headache and decreased concertation, etc., you can ask "what has happened recently?" or "what is going on in your life?" Then ask the patient how this is affecting her/him and what the most troubling thing about the problem is. This is followed by addressing how the patient is handling the situation and ending by showing empathy about what the patient is going through.

Dr.: I can see that all your symptoms including dizziness, fatigue and decreased concertation have started 3 months ago, what has happened recently? (Background)

Patient: My grandma is very sick and I am taking care of her.

Dr.: How does that make you feel? (Affect)

Patient (after a silence): angry and guilty.

Dr.: What is troubling you? What is it that makes you feel angry and guilty? (Trouble)

Patient: I am physically tired of taking care of her. I have to go to my school in the morning and take care of her in the evening. She has Alzheimer and she is kind of demanding. I love my grandma and I want to help my mother but sometimes I wish she passes away.

Dr.: This is not easy. How are you handling this situation? (Handle)

Patient: Not well. I am not able to study well. I feel jittery all the time.

Dr.: I can understand that this must be very difficult for a young person to take care of an old person while trying to continue one's studies (Empathy).

Patient: Exactly.

3. Rapport and Relationship Building

Rapport and relationship building is very important to put the patient at ease especially when PD patients might be reluctant to discuss their problems or show their emotions to the physician. There are many skills that allow the physician to build a better rapport and a trustworthy relationship with the patient. Below we will be looking at a number of such skills.

3.1. Breaking the Ice

Relationship building can start early on at the initiation of the session. When the patient walks in, the physician should stand up and salute her/him in a culturally appropriate way. Before asking for the chief complaint, the physician should engage in an informal chat to break the ice. This may help put the patient at ease. Breaking the ice is important for a patient who may have difficulty concentrating, as is the case with mental disorder patients or those not comfortable to discuss their problems. An example would be "I hope the traffic was acceptable on your way here," or "I noticed you were reading a book while waiting, hope you are enjoying it."

3.2. Patient Centered Approach

Adopting a patient centered approach and exploring the understanding of the patient and his/her beliefs will reduce the patient's anxiety, identify gaps in the knowledge of the patient and improve adherence to medication and illness outcomes. [18] There is no single approach or treatment that fits all. Understanding the patient's environment, community, family and socioeconomic status will help the physician to develop a better relationship with the patient and conclude with a management plan that the patient will adhere to. Trying to help beyond the clinic wall will further emphasize the idea that the physician cares about the patient as an individual.

> Dr.: I will solicit the help of the chairman of the math department if you have no problem with that.
>
> Patient (Delighted): What will you tell the chairman?
>
> Dr.: I will tell him that your poor performance is due to a disease and to give you a chance. I expect that after starting the treatment by 3-6

weeks your concentration will become better and this will reflect on your academic performance.

Patient: That would be great. I really appreciate it.

Dr.: I am going to prescribe Fluoxetine. Have you ever heard about this medicine?

Patient: Oh yes doctor. I don't want to take this medication. Most of my family members are taking Fluoxetine. I don't want to be like them. They are addicted to the medicine and have been taking it for many years.

Dr.: Let me explain more about the drug.........

4. Gathering Information and History Taking

4.1. Use of Open Ended Questions

Gathering information and history taking in PD patients can be quite challenging. Patients with mental health problems might lack concentration, have low self-esteem, and tend to minimize or maximize their problems; this affects negatively data gathering. [19] Open ended questions and silence allow patients to feel accepted by the doctor, to express their feelings, and reveal the required information. Physicians who use closed ended questions early in the consultation may miss the opportunity to have patients express their feelings which could deprive the physician from more clues to reach an appropriate diagnosis. Below is an example of open ended question.

Dr.: How can I help you?

Patient: I am confused and my grades are poor.

Dr.: (pauses for couple of seconds) May you elaborate more? {Directive open question}

Patient: I am a junior student in computer science. I am failing my math tests. This does not entitle me to continue postgraduate studies.

4.2. Summarization

Summarizing is one way to show the patient that the doctor was listening. It is also an opportunity that gives both the physicians and patients the chance to correct any misunderstanding. Summarization is extremely important in PD patients. For example, some anxious patients might tackle many items during the encounter and summarizing would be an excellent opportunity to focus the complaints. On the other hand, severely depressed patients might not volunteer lots of information and summarization in this case would be an opportunity for the physician to make sure he/she understood the problems of the patient. Ending the summarization with an open ended question allowing the patients to clarify or agree is highly essential.

> Dr.: I think I got a clear picture. My understanding is that your main problem is a mixed feeling of sadness and fear, decreased concentration, sleep problem, and lack of interest in activities you used to enjoy. You also feel uncomfortable when you meet a girl or you give a presentation. Is there anything you like to add?

5. Addressing Suicidal Status

All patients with mental health problems should be evaluated for suicidal ideation, plans, and attempts in the past and present. This can be done in several ways. Closed ended questions are more appropriate in this context. The physician may say "patients who do not cope well with stress may wish to sleep and not wake up at all. Do you have such a wish?" The physician might get an idea indirectly by asking the patient where s/he sees herself/himself a year ahead. Patients who respond positive to the first question or those who have no plans for the future need to be questioned if they have concrete plans to end their life.

> Dr.: Did the idea of hurting yourself cross your mind?
> Patient: In what way?
> Dr.: Like killing yourself.
> Patient: (adamant) No, no.

6. Addressing Sensitive Issues

Mental health illness is associated with comorbidities such as substance abuse and sexual dysfunction. When you want to ask personal questions deemed to be sensitive, prepare the patient for such a step. It is advised to assure the patient that the interview is confidential and define the situations in which the physician is obliged to breach the vow (suicidal or homicidal patients and under oath).

> Dr.: I like to tell you that whatever you tell me will be confidential. I am obliged to breech confidentiality if the information given to me jeopardizes the health of any person including yours. Now I like to ask some sensitive questions. Do you mind?
>
> Patient: Go ahead doctor.
>
> Dr.: Students at your age may like to experiment with drugs, have you done this?
>
> Patient: No
>
> Dr.: I need to ask you another sensitive question; how is your sexual drive?

7. Avoiding Unnecessary Investigations

7.1. Negotiation

Patients with mental disorders may be worried of having a serious problem like heart disease or malignancy. This is why they may insist on having several laboratory tests or procedures and may call their physician at odd times. Negotiation, if carried properly may abate unnecessary requests. When carried properly, the physical exam becomes an integral part of the negotiation process. A complete physical exam shows the patient that the physician entertained the possibility of a mental health problem after she/he has searched for physical problems.

> Dr.: As you see I carried a detailed physical exam; the exam is normal. Let me explain to you what your problem is. All your complaints are genuine and are caused by a chemical imbalance in your body.

Negotiation helps in recognizing the obstacles the patient perceives for the implementation of the plan, and provides solutions for them. Prerequisites for a successful negotiation are: (i) exploring, (ii) acknowledging, (iii) and addressing patient's beliefs and expectations. This is done in a respectful atmosphere. Failing to negotiate and reach a common understanding of the problem and its management results in unnecessary workup and poor compliance.

Dr:… I think your headache is caused by depression

Patient: Don't you think it is better to do MRI to the brain?

Dr.: Why do you want to do an MRI? (Explore)

Patient: I am worried about having a serious condition (deep sigh).

Dr.: What kind of serious condition? {Explore}

Patent: I am afraid to have a brain cancer.

Dr.: Why do you think you might have brain cancer? (Understand patient beliefs)

Patient: Cancers are common nowadays and I am worried about the decreased concentration.

Dr.: The headache has been for a while and I can understand that you are worried and afraid of having cancer. (Acknowledge and legitimize). However, the features of your headache are non-alarming and your physical examination, including the brain, is normal. The other associated symptoms like fatigue and memory loss, dizziness and the stress you are going through with your kids has led me to conclude that you might have depression.

Patient: But what if I have a brain cancer?

Dr.: How about this suggestion? I will give you a medicine for depression and see you in 4 weeks. If you do not feel better, we will reevaluate your headache. Is this fine with you?

Patient: Yes.

7.2. Explanation of the Mind-Body Relationship

In primary care settings, patients with depression or anxiety tend to emphasize more on the somatic symptoms such as fatigue, pain, insomnia. [20] They seek organic causes of their complaints and are not convinced that psychological distress can cause somatic complaint. Therefore, it is an important step to start with identification of the patients' concerns and acknowledgment that their symptoms are genuine. Physicians should explain why they are having the presenting symptoms by dwelling on the body mind relation. Physicians should avoid telling the patient that the symptoms are not important, that there is nothing wrong physically, or that the problem is in their head.

Visual aids enhance communication with patients (both literate and non-literate), enhance recall of spoken medical instruction and lead to long term retention of information. [21] A schematic drawing is of help (Figure). The diagram illustrates that the body functions are controlled by the brain through nerves that secrete chemicals and that the symptoms are caused by an imbalance in the amount of chemicals. Other chronic diseases such as diabetes mellitus could be used as an analogy. This model also helps to discuss the value of the medication(s) that will be prescribed as it (they) will help in adjusting the amount of chemicals in the body.

Dr.: I think your symptoms are caused by depression.

Patient: I know I might be stressed lately but I am feeling dizzy all the time. It is affecting my life.

Dr.: Diagnosis of depression does not mean that you are not feeling dizzy. You are truly feeling dizzy however the cause is not related to the ear or eye or any other organ but rather the results of imbalance of some substances in your nervous system.

Patient: silent with dissatisfied look in his eyes

Dr.: Let me explain further. Our body responds to the way we think and feel. When we are emotionally upset, there is some imbalance in some substances in the nervous system. The body will try to tell us there is something wrong with these substances by feeling different complaints like dizziness, headache, fatigue, stomach pain, etc. This is called the mind-body connection. (The doctor draws a brain-nerve connection, see figure) {Visual aids}.

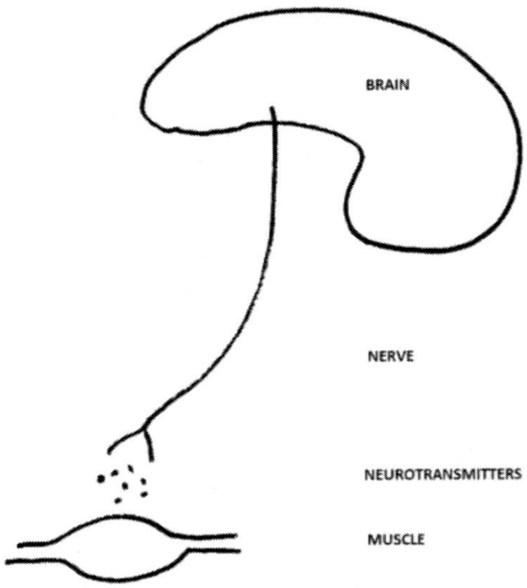

Figure. A schematic drawing used as educational material to explain the body-mind relationship to patients with mental health problems.

8. IMPROVE INITIATION AND ADHERENCE TO TREATMENT

8.1. Setting Expectations and Treatment Goals

It should be clear to the patient that selective serotonin inhibitors, TCAs, and others need approximately 4-6 weeks to have an adequate response. [22] Patients tend to stop the medication prematurely due to some untreated symptoms of depression like persistent low mood. [23] The physician may add that the first thing to improve is the sleep disturbance and that it would take longer for the mood to get better. If the patient's condition improves, she/he needs to know that the treatment needs to be continued for at least 4-6 months [22]. Setting reasonable expectation needs to be reemphasized in the treatment plan.

> Dr.: …Alprazolam was started to give you a quick relief. After three weeks, the amitriptyline is expected to control your sleep problem.
>
> Dr.: …I like you to know that we may not be able to get 100% improvement. The target is to make you function better; in your case the goal is that you graduate with an acceptable average.

8.2. Addressing Financial and Social Resources

Accommodating the financial and social resources of patients in the treatment plan will lead to better adherence. [24] Antidepressants have more or less similar efficacy but different side effect and tolerability profiles. Therefore, involving the patient in decision making and choice of the antidepressant is of utmost importance. The physician should always offer the patient the option between selective serotonin inhibitors (SSRI), tricyclic antidepressants (TCA), or other group of drugs after stating the cons and pros of each in case there is no contraindication. TCAs for instance should not be given in suicidal patients.

Tricyclic antidepressants still have a place in treating non-suicidal depression and anxiety in primary care. This is especially true when dealing with patients with limited financial resources and paying out of their pocket for the medicine. Adults and even older patients with no contraindications tend to tolerate TCA when the physician explains the common side effects before prescribing them. TCA need to be started at a low dose, and increased slowly to the desired dose.

It is important to emphasize that antidepressants do not result in addiction or tolerance as many patients are afraid to become dependent on TCA or SSRI. When stopping treatment the patient needs to know that this should be done gradually as many patients tend to stop the medication on their own when they start to feel better [25].

8.3. Follow Up Visits

Managing patients with mental disorders requires close follow up. Physicians should indicate when the follow up visit should occur. Many patients cannot afford frequent visits. In this situation, phone calls may ensure compliance. The phone call may be initiated by the physician or the patient. In the latter case, it is advisable to instruct the patient about the best time to call.

Giving cell phones to patients with mental disorders is controversial and depends on the preferences of the physician. Electronic mailing is another way of communication which may be less disturbing to the physician and more convenient to the patient. Patients need to be informed that electronic mailing is not secure or confidential. Patient/family members should be informed that urgent matters cannot be discussed using phone or emails and it should be clear to them where to go or who to contact in case of emergency.

Conclusion

The main challenge in communicating with psychologically distressed patients lies at the levels of gathering information and building rapport. Adopting an empathic and supportive attitude, focusing on open ended questions and adopting the bio-psycho-social model will help the patient "open up." Moreover, educating the patient about the symptoms and their causes using a schematic drawing might help in better adherence to medication and decreasing the stigma of the mental disorders.

References

[1] Tylee A, Gandhi P. The importance of somatic symptoms in depression in primary care. *Prim Care Companion J Clin Psychiatry* 2005;7(4):167-76.

[2] Clarkson P, Abendstern M, Sutcliffe C, Hughes J, Challis D. Identification and recognition of depression in community care assessments: impact of a national policy in England. *Int Psychogeriatr* 2012 Feb;24(2):261-9.

[3] Luppa M, Sikorski C, Motzek T, Konnopka A, Konig HH, Riedel-Heller SG. Health service utilization and costs of depressive symptoms in late life - a systematic review. *Curr Pharm Des* 2012;18(36):5936-57.

[4] Perez-Stable EJ, Miranda J, Munoz RF, Ying YW. Depression in medical outpatients. Underrecognition and misdiagnosis. *Arch Intern Med* 1990 May;150(5):1083-8.

[5] Siu AL, Bibbins-Domingo K, Grossman DC, Baumann LC, Davidson KW, Ebell M, et al. Screening for Depression in Adults: US Preventive Services Task Force Recommendation Statement. *JAMA* 2016 Jan 26;315(4):380-7.

[6] Kroenke K, Spitzer RL, Williams JB, Lowe B. The Patient Health Questionnaire Somatic, Anxiety, and Depressive Symptom Scales: a systematic review. *Gen Hosp Psychiatry* 2010 Jul;32(4):345-59.

[7] Malpass A, Dowrick C, Gilbody S, Robinson J, Wiles N, Duffy L, et al. Usefulness of PHQ-9 in primary care to determine meaningful symptoms of low mood: a qualitative study. *Br J Gen Pract* 2016 Feb;66(643):e78-e84.

[8] Gregory Vlastos. Slavery in Plato's thoughts. The Philosophical Review 1941;50(3):289-304.

[9] Accreditation Council for Graduate Medical Education. *ACGME Core Competencies.* 2012.

[10] Zolnierek KB, Dimatteo MR. Physician communication and patient adherence to treatment: a meta-analysis. *Med Care* 2009 Aug;47(8):826-34.

[11] Zandbelt LC, Smets EM, Oort FJ, Godfried MH, De Haes HC. Medical specialists' patient-centered communication and patient-reported outcomes. *Med Care* 2007 Apr;45(4):330-9.

[12] Stewart MA. Effective physician-patient communication and health outcomes: a review. *CMAJ* 1995 May 1;152(9):1423-33.

[13] Wun YT, Lam TP, Goldberg D, Lam KF, Li KT, Yip KC. Reasons for preferring a primary care physician for care if depressed. *Fam M*ed 2011 May;43(5):344-50.

[14] Craig TK, Boardman AP. ABC of mental health. Common mental health problems in primary care. *BMJ* 19 97May 31;314(7094):1609-12.

[15] Gomez G, Aillach E. Ways to improve the patient-physician relationship. *Curr Opin Psychiatry* 2013 Sep;26(5):453-7.
[16] Arikian SR, Gorman JM. A Review of the Diagnosis, Pharmacologic Treatment, and Economic Aspects of Anxiety Disorders. *Prim Care Companion J Clin Psychiatry* 2001 Jun;3(3):110-7.
[17] McCulloch J, Ramesar S, Peterson H. Psychotherapy in primary care: the BATHE technique. *Am Fam Physician* 1998 May 1;57(9):2131-4.
[18] Mauksch LB, Dugdale DC, Dodson S, Epstein R. Relationship, communication, and efficiency in the medical encounter: creating a clinical model from a literature review. *Arch Intern Med* 2008 Jul 14;168(13):1387-95.
[19] Gask L, Rogers A, Oliver D, May C, Roland M. Qualitative study of patients' perceptions of the quality of care for depression in general practice. *Br J Gen Pract* 2003 Apr;53(489):278-83.
[20] Wilhelm KA, Finch AW, Davenport TA, Hickie IB. What can alert the general practitioner to people whose common mental health problems are unrecognised? *Med J Aust* 2008 Jun 16;188(12 Suppl):S114-S118.
[21] Williams MV, Davis T, Parker RM, Weiss BD. The role of health literacy in patient-physician communication. *Fam Med* 2002 May;34(5):383-9.
[22] Carrie Armstrong. APA releases guideline on treatment of patients with major depressive disorder. *Am Fam Physician* 2008 Mar 15;83(10):1219-27.
[23] American Psychiatric Association. Practice guidelines for the treatment of patients with major depressive disorder. [Third edition]. 2010.
[24] Lynch JW, Kaplan GA, Salonen JT. Why do poor people behave poorly? Variation in adult health behaviours and psychosocial characteristics by stages of the socioeconomic lifecourse. *Soc Sci Med* 1997 Mar; 44(6):809-19.
[25] Demyttenaere K. Compliance and acceptance in antidepressant treatment. *Int J Psych Clin Pract* 2001;5(1):29-35.

BIOGRAPHICAL SKETCH

Name: **Basem Saab**

Address: Department of Family Medicine, American University of Beirut Medical Center, P.O. Box: 11 0236, Beirut- Lebanon

Current Position: Professor & program Director, Family Medicine Department, American University of Beirut Medical Center (AUBMC).

Education

Degree	Year	University/Examining body	Comment
Canadian Evaluating Examination.	Sept. 1988	The Medical Council of Canada	
Residency in Family Medicine	July 1984 – June 1987	American University of Beirut (AUBMC)	Qualification exam passed
MD	June 1984	AUBMC	
Internship in Internal Medicine	July 1983- June 1984	AUBMC	Good standing
BS	June 1979	American University of Beirut	Senior year with distinction

Research Activities

Interest in: Communication skills, ethics, social medicine, medical education, and minor surgery

64 publications in regional and international peer reviewed journals

Member of the International Advisory Board of the British Journal of General practice, International advisory board Journal of Bahrain Medical Society, and the Oman Medical Journal

Reviewed papers to 14 regional and international journals.

Publications over last 3 years

Ghadieh A, Saab B. Exercise in hypertensive patients: the evidence. *Can Fam Physician* 2015; 61: 233-239.

Agreus L, Saab B. International primary care snapshots: Sweden and Lebanon. *Br J Gen Pract* 2015; 65: 28-9.

Saab B, Ghadieh A. To not obscure the truth. *Br J Gen Pract* 2015; 65:91.

Saab B. The plight of Syrian refugees in Lebanon. . *Br J Genl Practi* 2014; 64: 94.

Saab B. When we justify apathy and homicide in Syria. *British Journal of General Practice* 2013; 63: 486.

Khoury L, Saab B, Musharrafieh U, Antoun J. Impact of a three days OSCE Workshop on Iraqi Physicians. *Fam Med* 2012; 44: 21-26.

Antoun J, Romani M, Saab B. Disclosure of Medical Error: Objective Structured Clinical Examination (OSCE). MedEdPORTAL; 2012. Available from: www.mededportal.org/publication/9226.

Saab B, Ghuloum S, Fayad Y. The classification of mental disorders in primary health care in the Arab region. *The Arab Journal of Psychiatry* 2012; 23 S:12-16.

Saab B. Medical Care: Elitism or Social Commitment. *British Journal of General Practice* 2012; 62:40-41.

Biographical Sketch

Name: **Jumana Antoun**
Affiliation: American University of Beirut, Lebanon

Education:

2011-2012; Masters in Health Informatics- Walden University
2001-2005; Specialist in Family Medicine - American University of Beirut
1997-2001; M.D., Medical School- American University of Beirut
1994-1997; B.S., Chemistry- American University of Beirut

Address: Department of Family Medicine, American University of Beirut, PO BOX 110236 Beirut, Lebanon

Research and Professional Experience:

Chair of the resident research committee

Involved in multiple research projects (received grants) (interest: communication skills, medical education and health informatics)

Core teaching faculty at the family medicine department

Member of the communication skills working group at Family Medicine department

Professional Appointments:

Assistant Professor, Family Medicine Department, American University of Beirut Medical Center

Publications Last Three Years:

1. Nasr, R., Antoun, J., Sabra, R., Zgheib, N.K. Interactive and collaborative learning in the classroom at the medical school: automated response systems and team based learning. LMJ. IN press.
2. Zoberi, K., Everard, K.M., Antoun, J. Teaching Chronic Pain in the Family Medicine Clerkship: Influences of Experience and Beliefs about Treatment Effectiveness. Family Medicine. IN press.
3. Antoun, J. Electronic mail communication between physician and patients: a review of challenges and opportunities. Family Practice, 2015. doi: 10.1093/fampra/cmv101. First published online: December 28, 2015
4. Antoun, J, Nasr, R, Zgheib, N.K. Use of technology in the readiness assurance process of team based learning: paper, automated response system or computer based testing. Computers in Human Behavior, 2015, 46:38-44.
5. Antoun, J, Hamadeh, G, Adib, S. What matters in the patients' decision to revisit the same primary care physician? LMJ, 2014, 62(4):198-202
6. Antoun, J, Romani, M., Johnson, A., Brock, C., Hamadeh , G. Balint seminars; the transatlantic experience through videoconference. Family Practice, 2014, 31(6):733-8. doi:10.1093/fampra/cmu065. Epub 2014 Oct 15.
7. Usta J, Feder, J, Antoun, J*. Attitudes towards domestic violence in Lebanon: a qualitative study of primary care practitioners. Br. J Gen Pract June 2014, 64: e313-e320; doi:10.3399/bjgp14X680077.

In: Communication Skills
Editor: Bridget L. Wright

ISBN: 978-1-63485-565-5

Chapter 3

COMMUNICATION NEUROSCIENCES FOR INTERPROFESSIONAL TEAMS IN HEALTH CARE

Carlo Lazzari[1] and Italo Masiello[2]
[1]Centre for Health Education,
Neuroeducation and Neuroleadership (CHENN),
Colechester, United Kingdom
[2]Department of Clinical Science and Education,
Karolinska Institutet, Södersjukhuset, Stockholm, Sweden

ABSTRACT

Recent developments in the neurosciences are offering an exclusive revision of all social and humanistic sciences. These also include psychology, counseling, mental health, and communication sciences. The idea that specific areas within the brain are activated during social interactions and communication is not recent. However, the brain has been found to record, react, and respond in unique and measurable ways when two or more people cooperate. In addition, prosocial behaviors, interpersonal communication, and teamwork also respond to a complex neurointegration of signals generated by the pairing of participants' brains, environment, and behavior. This chapter summarizes the major contributions that the neural sciences can provide to the understanding and improvement of prosocial communication and collaboration in healthcare and interprofessional teamwork. Prosocial communication for healthcare providers can be demanding and challenging. In fact, the participants in interprofessional activities should share proper communication skills to allow profitable interactions. Furthermore, they are also asked to integrate their behavior, attitudes, and expectations in order to promote the same communication milieu in the group. The neural mechanisms endorsing these adaptations are complex. However, recent advancements in the neurosciences allow an understanding of how the human brain functions in prosocial communication. Additionally, it is possible to stimulate group behavior that activates specific areas within the brain. This chapter will review major theories of neurocommunication intended as the application of the findings of neurosciences for the study of interprofessional communication and behavior in healthcare. All cerebral areas will be reconsidered in greater detail regarding their contribution to prosocial communication. Further details will be provided about instruments to study team interactions by recording group EEG or hyperscanning and neurocardiac studies on Heart Rate Variability (HRV) and Peripheral Oxygenation Variability (POV) during prosocial communication. In this chapter, we define communication neuroscience in interprofessional teamwork as the study of brain activities that determine prosocial communication, behaviors, skills, attitudes, and emotions of healthcare professionals involved in a collaborative practice. In this respect, the contribution of all cerebral areas is reconsidered as well as their influences on behaviors during interactive communication. This neurocommunicational perspective adds insight into the brain's functions that influence therapeutic and professional speech and listening. From here, neuroeducation can start with the intent to pair specific communication behaviors with the corresponding cerebral areas. The gain is a holistic and neurobehavioral theory of communication. The advantage is an understanding of that objective and neuroanatomical basis that generates and improves communication. The challenge is the creation of Neurocommunication Labs that allow the development of prosocial communication by understanding and training the social brain.

Keywords: neurosciences, neurocommunication, interprofessional communication skills

INTRODUCTION

Understanding how certain areas of the cerebral cortex function can also help clarify the behaviors correlated with those areas (Waldman et al., 2011). In the following sections, there is an explanation on how different brain areas can be studied and activated in order to promote better interprofessional communication and behavior (IPCB). Recent developments in neuroscience offer evidence-based "hard" science to help theorists of communication develop novel venues for explanations traditionally considered "soft" science (Ringleb & Rock, 2008). Furthermore, the development of neuroscience technology, like innovative mobile instruments to record brain activities and EEGs during social interactions, has further promoted the re-evaluation of concepts related to the soft sciences and communication. Neurocommunication deals with how people use their cortical areas to perform shared activities at their best and to promote a better quality of care for their clients.

The use of hard science and brain studies allows further insight into neuroactivities that are activated during social interactions and communication. Educating people to communicate better is also a way to explore and stimulate specific areas of their brain that regulate their emotions, speech, hearing, relationships, movements, memory, multi-tasking, and much more. It would be a limitation to consider only one of these aspects and to relate to them with a static model. Instead, the neurosciences show that peoples' minds are regulated by a flow of constant changes according to the circumstances where communication takes place.

Therefore, any measurement of a process, like communication, needs to detect the system as it changes over time (Battro, Fisher, & Léna, 2012). For example, the quality of prosocial communication is affected by several integrated factors, like the personality of the interacting people, their level of motivation to improve social exchanges, the level of tiredness or anxiety they are already experiencing, the time of the day, their interpersonal skills, and the state of attention and activation of their cortical areas. All these events can be explored with the help of soft and hard sciences' instruments merged into a unitary whole.

In some sense, there is a gain in the social mind that is not achievable in the individual mind. According to an anthropological point of view, what explains interactions are the independent circumstances of survival, such as shared situation and knowledge, not the subjective dimensions of morals, standards, sense, and individual aspirations (Barrett, 2015).

The challenge in creating a model for prosocial communication is, thus, to understand the intermediate passages that allow individual minds to act socially and to communicate in an integrated and synchronized way. In a certain sense, the concept of *intersection* is translatable into the notion of *cooperation*, definable as the condition in which two subjects must work together to obtain otherwise inaccessible prizes (Fujita et al., 2008).

In this chapter, *interprofessional teamwork* is seen as activity involving members of two or more occupations with paired competences in continued cooperative actions towards common goals (Barr & Low, 2013).

One hypothesis of this chapter is that an individual mind cannot live separately from other singular minds. At the same time, prosocial communication and mutual cooperation are not accidental events; indeed, they represent a natural occurrence of the individual development of each healthcare provider. Furthermore, it is hypothesized that a person is evolutionarily oriented to contextualize (be and behave in a certain social environment), socialize (either as cooperation or conflict), and communicate with peers via his/her own brain activities synchronously with others' brain events. These aspects carry implications for the social sciences, neuroeducation, and neuroeconomy, as conflicting communications and interactions may be a natural deviation from the norm of prosocial activities of the brain that also bring cooperation and prosocial communication.

A *modular view of mind* entails that the brain comprises a set of condensed systems containing information about how to orient itself in an uncertain and hostile social world (Kurzban & Aktipis, 2007). This definition also suggests that individual brains, as a subset of a social brain, also relate with each other according to the laws of chaos. In some respects, the effects of prosocial communication are not linear but have dynamic interferences due to the uncertainties of the interacting subjects in a team. One of these ambiguities in complex social systems involved in prosocial communication is the variation in the time of the collective variables, including knowledge, attitudes, and skills of each participant in a social interaction and communication episodes. For example, once cooperation proves to be beneficial for a group of healthcare providers to master difficult tasks, the individual brain incorporates a dynamic representation of the self-in-relation to others and others-in-relation to the self. Furthermore, this internal representation of the consequences of one's own communication with others activates certain areas of the prefrontal cortex.

Hence, the ability to form mental images or scenarios of the self-communicating-with-others, just before the actual interaction takes place, is a distinctive mark of mature social skills and prefrontal accomplishments. In fact, certain people, poor in mentalization processes, are not able to generate an internal scenario of their collective interactions and communication. This may also occur in a natural setting when healthcare workers are under stress and in a novel situation. Instead, mature cooperation and prosocial communication within small groups and interprofessional teams entails the ability to predict with a certain degree of probability *P* what the possible outcomes *O* are as a consequence of the interaction of the self-with-others (*swo*):

$$P(O)\ swo$$

without this intrinsic ability, a person would "communicate without thinking about the effect of the own communication on others," meaning that this person will not evaluate the effect that the own verbal and non-verbal messages have on the other people. This would only reduce empathic interactions while increasing elements of asocial communication. Moreover, as the social system is intrinsically variable, the laws of chaos also apply. Chaos is usually explained as a scientific characteristic of a dynamic system wherein time can either be a continuous or discrete variable (Bishop, 2015).

In mutually interacting, cooperating subjects, time is the major variable needed for changes in the neurocognitive system in order to allow mutual skills and prosocial communication. Similarly, according to time coordinates, social learning will promote the coordination of skills to allow the system (for example, a group of health professionals aiming to promote a better quality of care) to become more proficient by reducing errors and misinterpretations of environmental cues (e.g., symptoms of a patient admitted to Emergency) and interpersonal cues (e.g., collaborators' moods). From here, communication becomes more integrated with the exchange of empathic messages.

Furthermore, as this chapter will illustrate, a social brain is a natural occurrence in all public environments. Similarly, prosocial communication in interprofessional teams is not just the summative aspect of everyone's utterances. Consequently, the concept of the social brain and prosocial communication also applies to neurocommunication. An isolated healthcare provider who does not receive companionship and qualified support from peers could face serious challenges to his/her own professional integration and achievements. Social isolation has been viewed as a sign of a lack of collective skills to the point that a subject can no longer interact with peers (Frith & Frith, 2010). In addition, human beings learn to mentalize or to generate a theory of mind about other people by continuous interactions and communications with other persons. This skill—to predict with a low degree of error other people's thoughts, beliefs, actions, and messages—is called *mentalization*. It is a way of creating a theory of mind of what others might think, believe, communicate, and aim to do. Without this skill of mentalization, interpersonal interactions and prosocial communication would happen randomly and chaotically, with the tendency for everyone to generate misinterpretations, conflicts, and grey areas of communication, as hidden and social cues would be lost.

Therefore, social scientists feel that, when humans interact with others, humans must know something about others' psychology, such as their needs, understanding, and opinions, because this will help humans predict others' actions within the group (Frith & Frith, 2010). In order to mutually negotiate interprofessional communication, participants need to have a "theory of mind" of other participants in the group, that is, a *meta-representational* ability (Rochat & Ferreira, 2008). This means that, in order to initiate prosocial communication, each member of a team should have skills to represent mentally and to make speculations about what other participants in the interprofessional team know (the cognitive aspect of prosocial attitudes) or feel (the emotional part of prosocial attitudes) or how they plan to act (the behavioral component of prosocial beliefs).

One computational model representing communicational prediction is via the connection "if-then." This is symbolically represented by the arrow ⇒ indicating a predicate or antecedent, which causes another predicate or consequence. For example, "If I tell him so, then he reacts so." This could be simplified as: If x, then y, or $x \Rightarrow y$. Problems in utilizing mentalization are often found in people with autistic minds or pathologies of frontal lobes of the brain who habitually fail at social interactions because they are unable to predict others' minds, thoughts, feelings, desires, etc. Another logic symbol to represent the processes of mentalization is "therefore," ∴, which also indicates a consequence deriving from a premise. An illustration is someone thinking, "She is not talking (t) to me. Therefore, she is upset (u) with me." This is another process of guessing and mentalization, interchangeable with logic symbols:

"Not talking to me, therefore, upset":

$$\neg t \therefore u$$

And its opposite:

"Talking to me, therefore, not upset":

$$t \therefore \neg u$$

As a natural consequence, one should imagine a constant flow from an individual's self-talk and interaction (self-with-self as introspection) to group interaction and prosocial communication (self-with-other as extrospection). The term *extrospection* is defined by the Merriam-Webster on-line dictionary as "examination or observation of what is outside oneself, opposed to introspection." Consequently, the passage from the individual to the group, as action, and from the group to the individual, as re-action, sees a dynamic and evolutive process of interchanges in learning, action, attitudes, knowledges, skills, beliefs, and communication. Through the process of introspection, the subject evaluates the consequences (re-action) of the group's communication regarding the self. Through the process of extrospection, the subject acts on the group with his/her own self via verbal and non-verbal exchanges. The dynamic expressions then become:

Self⇔Others⇔Self…

Introspection⇔Extrospection⇔Introspection…

I ⇔ E ⇔ I

Therefore, in small-group dynamics and interprofessional communication, each participant evaluates the pros and cons of adapting his/her own communication style to the group's morals and ethos. At the same time, each healthcare professional weighs the pros and cons of promoting his/her own ideas to the group to probe whether it is convenient to communicate something about the self, about what is known, and about what should not be shared. As reported by neuroscientists, the brain is regularly shaped by self-reflection and by feedback from others as humans try to imitate others' minds during their exchanges (Clark & Dumas, 2015).

According to Vygotsky, the individual mind is represented by merging all the mentalized social interactions (registered into the individual mind) that the person has experienced in her/his life and that form her or his mind (Wertsch, 1985). Vygotsky is interested in "interpsychological" processes that are active in small groups of interacting and communicating people (Wertsch, 1985). Accordingly, communication models of the social brain arise through a consensual sharing of subjective truths. Hence, one way of constructing an "objective" reality is a collective (shared) one. This reflects the thinking of Kelly, the father of constructionism, who claimed:

> That is, knowledge of reality is not seen to be simply a matter of "taking a look" at the "facts" of the world in order to detect the degree of correspondence of those facts with our thoughts or beliefs (whether this be by direct perception or via representations). Rather, what we take to be a fact is assumed to be at least partly a function of our proactive outlook or framework of understanding (Stevens, 1998).

As a result, for a constructionist, there is no interest in focusing on an objective reality, but rather, on what constitutes a "better construction" of it (Stevens, 1998).

As social brain theories propose, human beings are not loner philosophers and they use communication to understand and survive in the world of ideas and facts. At the same time, communication would not exist out of a (pro)social context as there is always the need that at least two persons are into a reciprocal interaction. Indeed, as this chapter illustrates, knowledge belongs to *Homo Negotiatus*, as human beings are predisposed to contract and to debate the importance of objects and ideas until some accord is attained (Rochat & Ferreira, 2008). Therefore, the concept of truth is more a systemic debate that introduces and explains the interest in considering the social brain as the basis of prosocial communication. Perhaps interprofessional communication is a meta-theory of all theories very deeply linked to individual, social, emotional, environmental, cultural, and ethical conditions of the participants in a dialectical debate.

PREFRONTAL CORTEX AND PROSOCIAL COMMUNICATION

For a long time, the frontal lobes have been considered the center of volition, ethics, and planned behavior. The neuroassessment of their functions also carries indications of their behavioral component into interprofessional teamwork. For example, the Frontal Assessment Battery, or FAB (Dubois & Litvan, 2000; Slachevsky & Dubois, 2004), can be used to create guidelines to improve communication and interpersonal strategies led by the prefrontal cortex. For example, frontal lobes are important in the process of conceptualization and finding similarities, mental flexibility, programming, and resistance to interferences from the environment (Dubois et al., 2000; Slachevsky et al., 2004).

In order to promote prosocial communication in an interprofessional team, healthcare providers have to show skills in understanding others' feelings, emotions, and unspoken motives. This is usually referred to as the ability to have a Theory of Mind (ToM), intended as the capacity to recognize other people's mental state (Rowe et al., 2001). Frontal lobes are fundamental to the promotion of the ToM, as some pathologies affecting them make people unaware of social guidelines and the state of mind of others (Rowe et al., 2001). The improvement of the ToM is essential in order to implement one's own skills in IPCB. For example, professionals who show high social anxiety or affiliative needs might become highly or poorly sensitive to interpersonal cues. As a consequence, they are prone to misinterpret verbal and non-verbal messages proveening from their team, clients, and environment. The result is an impaired IPCB.

The frontal polar regions are necessary to the ToM for self-awareness, understanding the mental state of others, empathizing with them, and making appropriate social conclusions (Miller & Cummings, 2007). At the same time, people with an altered state of mind—under the effect of exogenous intoxication with illicit substances or affected by extreme anxiety, depression, tiredness, and fear—lose empathy, are mostly self-centered in their thoughts, and misinterpret social cues and communication. This can happen to healthcare providers under excessive stress and time constraints. Other times, with the aim to feel integrated with the group, several persons in a team start to talk and act in the same fashion as other team members. This can endanger self-identity and uniqueness while making communication styles redundant in each member of the team.

By utilizing FAB criteria, it is possible to implement a neuroprogramming of interprofessional communication with the following skills:

- Finding similarities: e.g., in what way is condition A similar to condition B? How can a nurse and doctor collaborate, assuming common interests and attitudes? In this case, shared tasks and goals will activate frontal-lobe neuroactivities.
- Mental flexibility: e.g., finding solutions that share the same characteristics. For example, how can the occupational therapist's skills be beneficial for the healthcare plan promoted by the nursing staff?
- Programming: being able to complete tasks in the correct order and in the right way. In this case, healthcare plans need to involve patients in their implementation. Doctors need to program in advance nurses' involvement in medical procedures before being able to achieve organizational outcomes in patients' health.
- Environmental autonomy: in order to communicate and interact properly in interprofessional teams, healthcare providers need to filter any interference to their jobs that is not strictly related to the duty performed at a certain moment. When nurses interact with patients, they should not be distracted by other ward routines.
- Motor functions: being capable of coordinating prosocial behaviors and communication to interact well with others and the environment.

Being capable of manipulating the social and professional environment to carry out tasks related to communication with patients as an interprofessional team.

- Higher-order functions: creativity and enlightenment. Finding new solutions for old problems. Discovering original venues and inventing new things, procedures, and solutions to work collaboratively within a team. Finding collective solutions to patients' health problems.
- Planning: the act or process of making or carrying out plans; specifically, the establishment of goals, policies, and procedures for social or economic utility (Merriam-Webster Dictionary); being able to predict possible future scenarios during interpersonal communication. Utilizing one's own social mind to understand what happens after verbal and non-verbal messages are shared in an interpersonal context. Predicting the consequence of one's own communication with those involved in the interpersonal activities.
- Reasoning: "The process of thinking about something in a logical way in order to form a conclusion or judgment" (Merriam-Webster Dictionary). Utilizing procedural guidelines in order to promote professional communication with patients.
- Impulse control: being able to delay immediate reactions and distress for the good of interprofessional team communication. Being capable of controlling emotions to improve team communication. Delaying immediate gratification (e.g., an authoritarian communication style) for the sake of prosocial communication (e.g., an affiliative communication style).
- Memory: "The power or process of remembering what has been learned" (Merriam-Webster Dictionary). Becoming self-reflective and learning from one's own errors or achievements in IPCB.
- Spontaneity: utilizing open communication styles, frank prosocial verbal and non-verbal styles and postures, and the avoidance of undisclosed meanings for open communication.
- Problem solving: providing the self and others with proper communication cues and information (verbal, non-verbal, written, electronic, etc.) in order to succeed in shared activities, leading to customer satisfaction.
- Initiation: skills and attitudes to promote prosocial communication styles and the avoidance of passive attitudes towards IPCB.

- Judgement: the ability to distinguish areas of distress caused by faulty communication styles and understanding their impact on the well-being of teams and clients.
- Social behavior: mostly related to recognizing the rules of interpersonal engagement, support, and empathy for what concerns interprofessional teams.

THE CORPUS CALLOSUM AND MULTI-TASK NEUROCOMMUNICATION

Communicating properly requires constant attention to a multifaceted array of factors, including the self, the others, and the environment. Recent studies reappraise the utility of the corpus callosum in multi-task performances and in preconceived interpretations of its functions. For example, it has been found that there is no substantial difference in the size and shape of the corpus callosum in both genders (Bishop & Wahlsten, 1997). However, the splenium encloses more fibers in females than males, and in rats, the mid-sagittal area is larger in females than males (Clark, Boutros, & Mendez, 2010).

Language normally involves information handling between both cerebral hemispheres. For example, people who are able to master more than their native language since infancy show a larger posterior midbody midsagittal area, which is linked to an increase in the number of connections created between right and left hemispheres (Coggins et al., 2004).

If this is confirmed, afterwards, it becomes interesting to promote a neurocognitive change of prosocial and interprofessional communication by exposing learners and healthcare providers to environments where two or more languages are spoken. For example, this can be achieved by promoting international exchanges of healthcare providers who are then introduced to shared teamwork, which happens at the Karolinska interprofessional training center.

Multi-tasking can also be implemented by exposing learners to diverse responsibilities in an array and helping them interact and communicate by utilizing a shared protocol of tasks. Finally, the self-assessment of neurophysiological variables (e.g., heart rate variability, respiratory rate, ECG, and EEG) during interprofessional activities should implement multi-tasking and cerebral connections. A paper published by the National Organization for Disorders of the Corpus Callosum (2016) mentions that people with pathologies of the corpus callosum with partial or total agenesis are unaffected by the opinions and states of mind of other people, misinterpret social signals (e.g., they cannot interpret non-verbal messages or tone of voice), and lose an understanding of their own behavior, social complications, and interpersonal encounters. Caoa et al., (2013) have found that children with Attention Deficit and Hyperactive Disorder (ADHD) have macro- and micro-structural abnormalities in the corpus callosum.

Prosocial and multi-tasking neurocommunication include:

- Developing multilingual skills in a multi-ethnic environment.
- Learning how to communicate in teams populated by international professionals.
- Learning a second or third language and applying these skills in a team that shares these languages.
- Interacting in multiprofessional teams by understanding and sharing jargon-free verbal cues.

The Reptilian Brain and Unbiased Communication

Prosocial behavior and communication entails efforts to understand others' frames of mind and to overcome egocentric interpretations of social reality. This is usually referred to as *allocentric* skills, which are characterized as the ability to center attention on interpersonal cues and an objective social milieu more than on a subjective and egocentric social space. This space can be physical, like the world of things, but also social, like others, small groups, and interprofessional teams. The hippocampus (reptilian brain) is essential to the representation of an allocentric space where objects are symbolized in relation to other objects (but not to the self) (Nauman et al., 2015). For example, if a doctor tells a nurse that the patient has a blocked artery in the legs without specifying, for example, the term "DVT," he is assuming from a personal perspective, but not from the allocentric perspective of the nurse, that she knows what he is mentioning.

The reptilian brain is, thus, basic for the encoding of relationships among numerous environmental entities (*place learning*) (Nauman et al., 2015). Becoming disentangled by one's own subjective space and being able to locate the self in an objective and interpersonal environment are essential skills for prosocial communication. Learners in interprofessional teams should, therefore, be trained in constructing messages from an allocentric point of view to reduce the risk of assuming that others in the group share their own frame of reference, knowledge, and beliefs. For example, without this capacity, young turtles from hatched eggs would never be able to make their way back to the sea if they referred themselves to an egocentric space composed of dunes along the shore surrounding them. They need to orient themselves, and in doing so, include diverse cues like the sky, shadows, shapes, etc.

The Parietal Lobes, Writing, and Congruent Communication

Parietal lobes are involved in the coordination of movements required for writing, while pathologies in the parietal lobes result in the absence of graphical skills, called *agraphia* (Brownsett & Wise, 2010). One can assume that parietal lobe functioning is necessary for all forms of communication in the healthcare setting that include writing, like entries in electronic systems, patients' assessments, composing letters, and written communications to colleagues. In addition, parietal lobes are also essential in the manipulation of numerical data (like vital signs, dosages of medications, understanding quantities, and disparities in amounts). According to scientists, left parietal lobes are involved in the extraction and comparison of learned numeric data; on the other hand, right parietal lobes are involved in the symbolic manipulation of numeric figures (Cappelletti et al., 2010). Parietal lobes are also essential in the recall of autobiographical memories (Berryhill et al., 2007).

The use of biographical memories, especially for the self-with-others, is essential in order to structure historical communications. These emerge from the consolidation of several communication events related to the self-with-others that occurred in the past. These historical events require a memory of what is said, how it is said, and to whom. In fact, proper communication is not a process simply related to the here and now. Particularly evident in the mental-health professions, healthcare providers need to memorize the communication events they had with their clients (e.g., a psychotherapist, a counselor) and be in tune with previous verbal exchanges. This skill is necessary in order to avoid discrepancies in what is told in the past and in the present. This communication memory is also essential in order to be coherent with oneself-towards-colleagues ("Yesterday you told me this! Today, you're saying something different!") and the self (e.g., communication coherence). This cognitive and biographical coherence is a vital quality in interprofessional teams.

THE TEMPORAL LOBES AND COMMUNICATION MEMORY

The dorsolateral temporal lobe plays a central role in auditory and speech recognition, while it also appears to be involved in autism (Clark, Boutros, & Mendez, 2010). The temporal lobes (TLs) are necessary for attributing meaning to humans' experiences in the world involving the integration of data from sensory, motor, and verbal experiences (Hoffman, Evans, & Lambon Ralph, 2014). In other words, conceptual representations are stored as verbal and non-verbal information in the anterior temporal lobes (Bonnì et al., 2015). Therefore, it can be assumed that the recollection of communication events is stored in the TLs, which also provide meaning to these episodes by integrating the auditory and verbal experiences linked to them.

Therefore, TLs have mostly been linked to the following communication skills:

- Understanding of language.
- Behavioral, motor, and social components (people with temporal lobe epilepsy display changes in their personalities).
- Memory.
- Hearing: primary and association.
- Linking past and present sensory and emotional experiences with a continuous self.

The communication skills that characterize and require the activations of the temporal lobes are:

- Empathic listening and attention to what is told or heard.
- Memorization of communication events and merging of different communication experiences into a meaningful theory of others.
- Competence in understanding and providing a meaning to spoken language and expressed emotions of others.

- Organization of verbal and non-verbal messages from others into meaningful information together with the memorization of these concepts and prosocial communications.

Medial temporal lobes (the parahippocampal gyrus and hippocampus) have a function in the recognition memory of faces and scenes independent of the observational perspective (Taylor, Henson, & Graham, 2007).

From the neurobehavioral functions of TL, one can derive some ideas about prosocial communication in interprofessional teams:

- Communication events are not distinct events of the self-with-others. Instead, a construction of meanings during interactions with others is necessary to the achievement of prosocial communication. These processes require the TL activation of mnemonic traces of social events.
- Prosocial communication in interprofessional teams is a distinctive event that is different from simple speech and hearing. Instead, a fine integration of hearing and speech centers is important in order to achieve better quality in verbal and non-verbal communication.
- Recall and communication are not two separate events. Instead, in order to produce acceptable prosocial dialogue and unified verbal and non-verbal behavior, humans have to mix different segments of these social interactions:
    - A recollection of any interactions with other people in the same team and understanding of the meanings deriving from the outcomes of these interactions.
    - A semantic memory of the communication units utilized that were successful in the achievement of prosocial behaviors.
    - An approximate prediction of the outcomes of any ongoing communication in the team based on stored scenarios of any previous communication event with the same people or similar people, in the identical environment or a similar environment, in the same conditions or in similar conditions.

Heart-Brain Connections and Emotional Neurocommunication

The importance of the heart in emotional regulations of behavior has been recently confirmed by neuroscientists investigating the neuroanatomy of this organ. Current studies show that the human heart is intrinsically and bilaterally connected with the brain to the point that a mutual influence is also being hypothesized. For the sake of the communicational neurosciences, emotional, behavioral, and physiological factors can affect the heart and vice versa. As a consequence, it becomes imperative that prosocial communication is done with the right state of heart and mind. For example, the amount of blood that reaches the brain is controlled by the heart, and there is evidence that any abnormality of brain perfusion will cause cognitive impairments (Ritz, van Buchem, & Daemen, 2013). Historically, emotional stress has been considered a noxious agent on hearts, leading to possible arrhythmias and myocardial infarction. Recent discoveries at the University of California, Berkeley, also provide evidence that chronic stress produces alterations in the brain, perhaps due to an increase of myelin and white matter in some areas of the brain and an alteration of the messages between areas of the brain (Sanders, 2014). There are also studies reporting that severe psychological stress predisposes one to Alzheimer's dementia (Tsolaki et al., 2009), while constant exposure to stressful life events can lead to later cognitive dysfunctions (Greenberg et al., 2014).

By looking at these studies, one can hypothesize that a traumatic communication can generate long-lasting stress. At the same time, there might be direct effects upon the brain that, either altered by the emotional consequences of the pathological communication or by the neurotoxicity of the stress, will jeopardize the encoding and decoding neuromechanisms at the origin of prosocial communication. For example, listening to rebuffs will alter the heart-brain neurophysiology to the point that a person might respond with cardiac arrhythmias, dizziness, confusion, or some mild to severe behavioral changes. At this point, the brain can influence the heart and vice versa. The final effect is that a person who has created a mnemonic trace of the morbid communication will not be able to coordinate the proper brain functions to communicate clearly with that person who is threatening her or him. In other words, pathological communications in hospitals or wards can alter the delicate mind-brain mechanisms that allow a person, say, a victim of bullying or authoritarian communication, to restore the proper balance in the neurophysiological centers for prosocial communication. As a consequence, because of the mnemonic trace of the traumatic relation with others, a person who is under stress and anxiety for interpersonal reasons develops lasting neurophysiological symptoms (e.g., palpitations, irritable bowel syndrome, etc.) that impede the fine neuroregulation of heart-brain-speech centers (Figure 1). She/he might mumble in the same stressful conditions; other times, he/she might decide not to talk at all because of cardiac palpitations when facing tense rapports, e.g., a despotic colleague or a tyrannical manager.

Research shows that, if a relaxed brain is necessary to regulate the heart's rhythm, the opposite happens during stress and anxiety. For example, "heart coherence" is the organization of heartbeats under brain meditation with reciprocal influence and synchronized activities between EEG alpha rhythm and cardiac rhythm (Kim et al., 2013). The authors of this chapter, who have observed social exchanges in their neurocardiac lab, also show that people interacting in a group have synchronized heart-rate variabilities (HRV) (Figure 4). This reinforces the idea that people acting in small groups and involved in prosocial communication have coordinated neurophysiological variables, including EEG, Heart Rate Variability (HRV), Peripheral Oxygenation Variability (POV), and Respiratory Rate Variability (RRV).

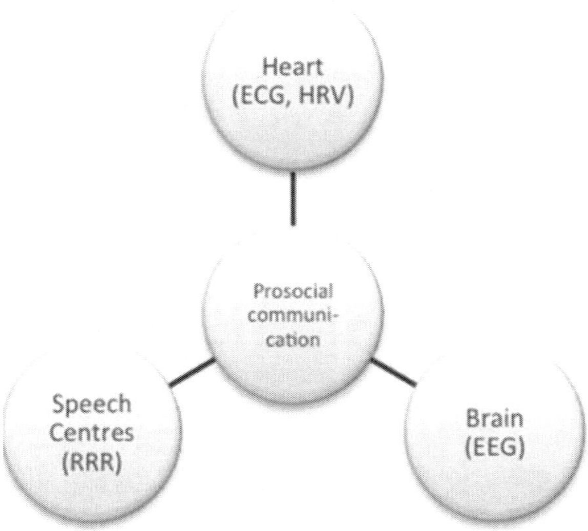

Figure 1. The integration of Heart Rate Variability (HRV), ECG, EEG, and speech centers involved in Registering, Remembering and Reacting (RRR) to visual and auditory signals generates the neurophysiological basis for prosocial communication.

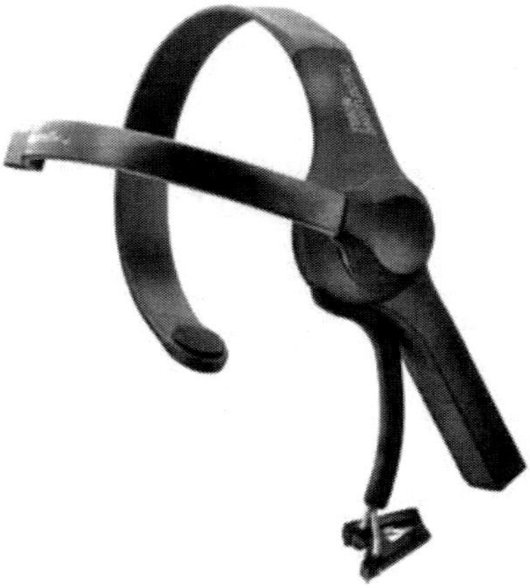

Figure 2. Headset from Neurosky® portable EEG. The disposal of several softwares and apps makes it user friendly for recording brain activities of people involved in a meangful conversation.

These findings also support the discovery of the "brain in the heart" (Armour, 2007). In fact, the human heart has been found to have its own intrinsic and independent nervous center, a form of intrathoracic neurons in the heart with afferent and efferent neurons free from the control of the brain (Armour, 2007).

These data would endorse the hypothesis that the synchronization of heart-brain-neurocommunication activities has robust justification supported by the neurophysiological correlation between these neurosystems. Everything applied in prosocial interactions shows that people communicate within a group with their brain, heart, and speech centers. Furthermore, the synchronized activities of these systems are the origin or consequence of coordinated emotions that produce the final verbal and non-verbal communication. As previously seen, stress and emotions can alter the neurobalance of the brain-heart-speech centers (HBS). At this point, prosocial communication is no longer possible. For example, chronic interpersonal stress and conflicts generate permanent memories of these interactions. Afterward, a person will show automatic hyperactivation of the HBS axis. Communication in a group will become difficult with many neurophysiological reactions, like palpitations, altered tone of voice, increased respiratory rate, abnormal pace of speech, flushing, and interrupted flow of spontaneous speech. The HBS is no longer synchronized, and the clarity in expressing the self to others will show evident flaws.

MIRROR NEURONS AND EMPATHIC COMMUNICATION

Mirror neurons are the neural basis for a direct and semantic link between communicating people. Simultaneously, they allow the actions of each person to be clear to other people without cognitive intermediation (Rizzolatti & Craighero, 2004). Based on this neurophysiological aspect, one can assume that prosocial communication implies some nervous mechanism that is only partly under the direct control of participants in a communicative exchange. This can be seen, for example, when two persons communicate. It is likely that, at a certain point, if they are open enough to each other, they will display the same gestures, an identical tone and rate of speech, and even similar accents. This dance of feelings helps people register what emotions are experienced during their communication with others. In addition, via the action of mirror neurons, people in a team with true empathic skills will be able to orient themselves and understand what others are experiencing, feeling, or even thinking, although this is not openly manifested during the prosocial communication. A subtle mechanism has tuned the neurocommunication of this team like musicians in the same orchestra. With a detailed assessment of their EEGs, one can even see that they tend to display the same level of attention, anxiety, calm, or distress if they are in tune with each other (Figure 3).

Imitation occurs as an action of mirror neurons. People might first observe skilled others while communicating. Thereafter, they start to copy what they see and hear. Finally, people start to use communication as an automatic process. Composite imitation combines the aptitude to identify another's action as a set of recognizable movements with the capacity to use this detection to duplicate the performance (Arbib, 2011). Therefore, mirror neurons expedite the aptitude to understand the actions and emotions of others. In fact, the observation of facial expressions of other people triggers the observer's limbic system (specifically, a network inclusive of mirror neurons, insula, and limbic areas), producing in the observer the same emotions of the people observed (Iacoboni, 2009).

Other authors are skeptical about the presence of mirror neurons, the presence of which has been directly demonstrated in monkeys in the F5 motor area of the brain and indirectly in humans (Harriet, 2015). Mirror neurons have been advocated as being at the basis of the Motor Theory (MT) of speech perception, suggesting that we recognize speech by recreating the motor gestures that produced those sounds (Harriet, 2015).

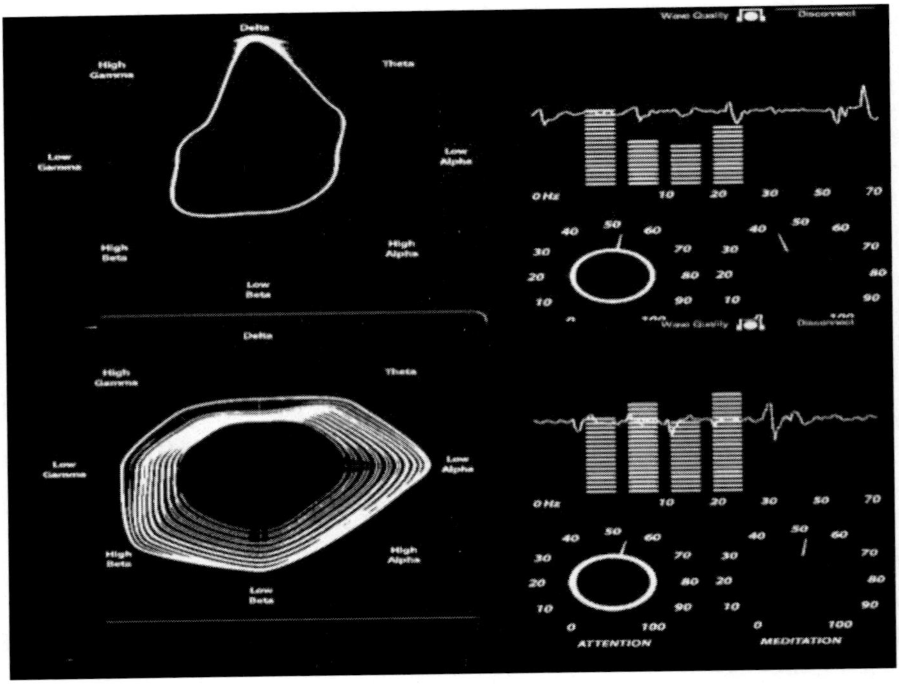

Figure 3. Two EEG traces from two healthcare professionals interacting. The two 'Attention' meters show the same level of attention in both persons.

This last neural mechanism for empathy suggests that prosocial communication is a subconscious integration of people's proclivity to accommodate their own emotions according to the imitation and understanding of others' emotions. This mechanism, as we have seen, is under the control of mirror neurons. In addition, by learning to decipher their own emotions when involved in interprofessional activities, healthcarers can anticipate the emotions of other people in their team. The major skill in prosocial communication is thus an improvement of this neuronal mechanism for empathy promoted by mirror neurons.

NEUROCOMMUNICATION LAB

The Neurocommunication Lab (NCL®) designed by the authors of this chapter (Lazzari, Masiello, & Shoka, 2016) is a physical space provided with multiple neurophysiological instruments (EEG, ECG, Pulseoxymeter, etc.) to record the activities of people involved in mutual interactions and communication. The confluence of multi-channeled registrations of neurophysiological parameters of participants within interprofessional groups is longitudinally recorded. Each subject of the team is connected via wires to a pulseoxymeter and portable EEG that interface with a computer. The simultaneous registration of Heart Variation Rate (HVR), Peripheral Oxygenation Variability (POV), and EEG allows the measurement of neurosocial data of people engaged in prosocial communication. In addition, the objective measurement of simultaneous EEGs (Figure 3) of people interacting in a group has been defined as *hyperscanning* (Babiloni & Astolfi, 2014). This technique has been extended in the Neuroleadership Lab (NLL) to include the simultaneous recording of multiple neurophysiological variables, including EEG (hyperscanning) Heart Rate Variability (HRV), Peripheral Oxygenation Variability (POV), and Respiratory Rate Variability (RRV) (Figure 4). Raw data are collected as numerical values and utilized for statistical evaluation.

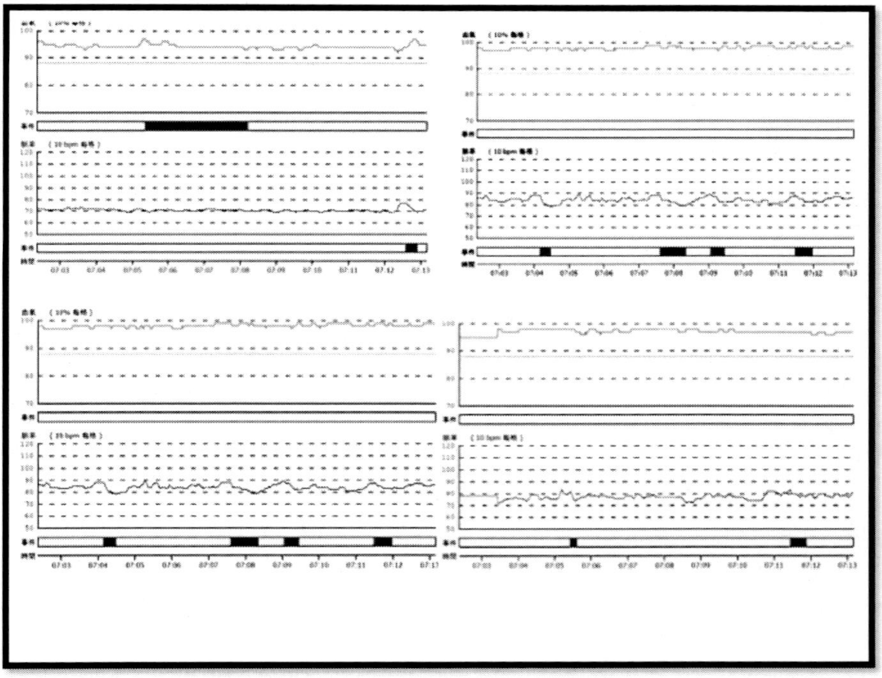

Figure 4. Three healthcare workers communicating with a patient (upper left). There is some sychrony and congruity in the heart rate (lower traces) and peripheral oxygenation (upper traces).

In an experimental condition, each person in the NLL group takes the lead on a selected scenario and seeks the collaboration of other team members. The neuroemotional and consensual parameters are then recorded as group neuroleadership variables. The two major outcomes are the *Neurointeracting Group (NIG)* and the *Neurodisjointed Group (NDG)*. In the NIG, there are similar and synchronized variations (consensual increase or decrease in neurophysiological variables and activations of similar cortical areas) during interactive communications. The opposite happens in NDG. For example, if a leader feels confident in communicating a healthcare plan, then the instruments will record a state of relaxation with low HRV, POV, and alpha EEG rhythm in that person and others. However, if the team feels angry about this project, then all the neurophysiological parameters will show this. The discrepancy between leader and team neurovariables will generate an NDG, and the team will be considered desynchronized for what concerns empathic communication.

The development of portable EEGs (Figure 2) mostly from Neurosky® and Emotiv® has allowed the registration of brain activities of people involved in meaningful and prosocial communication. This is to say that states of attention, meditation, alertness, and concentration during interpersonal communication can be recorded consensually. This allows dynamic neurofeedback with the optimization of participants' brain activities, mainly their attention/meditation polarity during their prosocial communication.

NEUROEDUCATION IN COMMUNICATION SKILLS

The concept of educating people to improve their communication skills has always been the goal of educationalists. However, the new field of neuroeducation is opening novel venues in understanding how this can be done with the guideline of neurosciences. There are some ethical issues surrounding the study of the interactions between neurosciences and education posed by the risk of using invasive instruments to detect brain activities of the interacting people, mostly Magnetic Resonance Imaging (MRI) (Maxwell & Racine, 2012). At the same time, there are several noninvasive instruments that can provide real-time contextual recordings of the neurophysiological variations of people involved in a prosocial exchange, such as those seen in the Neurocommunication Lab. Instead, it is more likely that resistances or misunderstandings can arise from those who have no sufficient background in the neurosciences to embrace the potential benefits of this science to tackle everyday problems in education.

However, if someone can communicate by using all the functions of the cortical areas, then one can say that there has been attention to how communication can be performed in a holistic way, with the guideline of the hard sciences and with the knowledge of how the brain elaborates personal and social cues for communicating in groups. The case of a person in an interprofessional team who can perform his/her own task to communicate with colleagues in a clear fashion, to find an empathic posture with clients, and to listen to all environmental cues illustrates an integrated approach to neurocommunication. This could be interpreted, for example, as the use of a frontal prosocial posture with clients, the application of a multi-tasking corpus callosum, like the attitude in having interactions with different colleagues at the same time, and the control of auditory cues to select environmental sounds and to filter what is important in dealing with contextual challenges. Therefore, the neurosciences help in interpreting prosocial communication as a natural occurrence of well-coordinated individual minds. This field of research also allows the focusing of scientists' attention on performances and outcomes of interacting people and on promoting better communication via targeted actions on specific cerebral areas.

When parents direct their children with prosocial behaviors, involuntarily, they are reinforcing prefrontal controls of impulses. When a physiotherapist helps people with limited functions to activate cognate muscular groups, they are reinforcing neuronal integrations in the motor areas. It would be a loss if neuroscience were disjoined by any other element affecting brain alertness like tiredness after long shifts, which impairs prosocial communication, or the impact of interpersonal distress, which disturbs the proclivity to activate prosocial behaviors. Environmental events do affect bodily physiology, even if simply in the variation in heart rate or lung oxygenation. If one respects the complexity of the interactions of environment, body, and brain, then any distressing or activating external events do carry a certain impact on physiological responses, personal well-being, and prosocial attitudes in communication. For example, people in the early hours of a shift do show different patterns of communication compared to late hours of shifts after a tiresome day.

These and other examples reinforce the concept that communication, and mainly prosocial communication, require the coordination of different mental and brain processes. Initially, the concepts that characterize a discourse will be organized into the minds of communicating people. Then, people involved in collective communication need to become synchronous with their neurophysiological and neuroemotional parameters in order to activate prosocial communication. Afterwards, when all these factors have been satisfied, shared meanings are generated as the coordination of mental processes that control social language and interactions. Although in this chapter, single brain areas have been indicated as controlling specific aspects of prosocial language, at this moment, there is no conclusive remark that language can be separated into sub-categorical events. Rather, all neurocognitive and neuroemotional actions that generate a prosocial communication are interrelated. As Schnelle (2010) suggests, the brain has no dominant workstation and no practical separation in representation arrangements, and there is no identifiable structure for symbol grouping, partings, or reorganizations. Schnelle (2010) comments:

> The available structures of the world do not exist independently of our mind/brain/body's organization generated in a mutual cooperation and communication among a social group of people (p. 154).

CONCLUSION

In this chapter, the authors have examined different neurocognitive aspects of collective and interprofessional communication within the healthcare system. The authors are aware that this is not a common way of studying this aspect; however, they have tried to provide theoretical support of the processes that undergo prosocial communication. The application of neurophysiological recordings during prosocial communication seems to confirm the interplay of different and subjective elements merged into meaningful prosocial communication. Language is the way in which humans' social brain expresses itself. Prosocial communication is thus part of the social brain. People are synchronized when they communicate with their colleagues, patients, or anyone else present in the social and healthcare scenario.

Healthcare professionals collaborating with synchrony and synergy achieve acceptable prosocial communication. This will then lead to a better quality of care. Other facts enter the social equations of prosocial communication in interprofessional teams in health care. Supporting this complex dynamic are our brain system and the cerebral cortex. Evolution has then provided our social brain with distinctive features and with the ability to have the advantage of predicting communication outcomes before the actual events happen. Furthermore, the skill to mentalize and to empathize are supported by mirror neurons, while the direction of communication and information is regulated by instincts and emotions according to the group outcome when involved in social communication.

References

Arbib, M. A. (2011). From mirror neurons to complex imitation in the evolution of language and tool use. *The Annual Review of Anthropology, 40*, 257–273.

Armour, J. A. (2007). The little brain on the heart. *Cleveland Clinical Journal of Medicine, 74*(1), S48–S51.

Babiloni, F., & Astolfi, L. (2014). Social neuroscience and hyperscanning techniques: Past, present and future. *Neuroscience and Biobehavioral Reviews, 44*, 76–93.

Barr, H., & Low, H. (2013). Introducing interprofessional education. Fareham: CAIPE. Retrieved from: http://caipe.org.uk/silo/files/introducing-interprofessional-education.pdf.

Barrett S. (2015). *Anthropology: A student's guide to theory and method* [e-book]. Toronto: University of Toronto Press.

Battro, A. M., Fisher, K. W., & Léna, P. F. (2012). Introduction: Mind, brain, and education in theory and practice. In: Battro, A. M., Fisher, K. W, Léna, P. F. (Eds.), *Educated brain* (2nd ed.). Cambridge: Cambridge University Press.

Berryhill, M. E., Phuong, L., Picasso, L., Cabeza, R., & Olson, I. R. (2007). Parietal lobe and episodic memory: Bilateral damage causes impaired free recall of autobiographical memory. *The Journal of Neuroscience*, *27*(52), 14415–14423.

Bishop, K. M., & Wahlsten, D. (1997). Sex differences in the human Corpus Callosum: Myth or reality? *Neuroscience & Biobehavioral Reviews, 21*(5), 581–60.

Bishop, R. (2015). Chaos. In: *The Stanford Encyclopedia of Philosophy*. Retrieved from: http://plato.stanford.edu/archives/win2015/entries/ chaos/>.

Bonnì, S., Koch, G., Miniussi, C., Stampanoni Bassi, M., Caltagirone, C., & Gainotti, G. (2015). Role of the anterior temporal lobes in semantic representations: Paradoxical results of a cTBS study. *Neuropsychologia, 76*, 163–169.

Brownsett, S. L. E., & Wise, R. J. S. (2010). The contribution of the parietal lobes to speaking and writing. *Cerebral Cortex, 20*, 517–523.

Caoa, Q., Li Suna, L., Gongc, G., Lvd, Y., Caoa, X., Shuaia, L., Zhud, C., Yufeng Zangd, Y., & Wanga, Y. (2010). The macrostructural and microstructural abnormalities of corpus callosum in children with attention deficit/hyperactivity disorder: A combined morphometric and diffusion tensor MRI study. *Brain Research*, *1310*, 172–180.

Cappelletti, M., Lee, H. L., Freeman, E. D., & Price, C. J. (2010). The role of the right and left parietal lobes in the conceptual processing of numbers. *J. Cogn. Neurosci.*, *22*(2), 331–346.

Clark, D. L., Boutros, N. N., & Mendez, M. (2010). *The brain and behavior: An introduction to behavioral neuroanatomy.* Cambridge: Cambridge University Press.

Clark, I., & Dumas, G. (2015). Toward a neural basis for peer-interaction: What makes peer-learning tick? *Frontiers in Psychology, 6*(28), 1–12.

Coggins 3rd, P. E., Kennedy, T. J., & Armstrong, T. A. (2004). Bilingual corpus callosum variability. *Brain and Language, 89*, 69–75.

Dubois, B., & Litvan, I. (2000). The FAB: A frontal assessment battery at bedside. *Neurology*, *55*(11), 1621–1626.

Frith, U., & Frith, C. (2010). The social brain: Allowing humans to boldly go where no other species has been. *Philosophical Transactions of the Royal Society B*, *365,* 165–175.

Fujita, K., Kuroshima, H., Hattori, Y., & Takahashi, M. (2008). Social intelligence in Capuchin monkeys. In: Itakura, S., & Fujita, K. (Eds.), *Origins of the Social Mind: Evolutionary and Developmental Views*, Tokyo: Springer.

Greenberg, M. S., Tanev, K., Marin, M-F., & Pitman, R. K. (2014). Stress, PTSD, and dementia. *Alzheimer's & Dementia*, *10*, S155–S165.

Harriet, H. (2015). The use and abuse of mirror neurons. A review of "The Myth of Mirror Neurons: The real neuroscience of communication and cognition" by Gregory Hickok. *www.skeptic.com, 20*(2), 51.

Hoffman, P., Evans, G. A. L., & Lambon Ralph, M. A. (2014). The anterior temporal lobes are critically involved in acquiring new conceptual knowledge: Evidence for impaired feature integration in semantic dementia. *Cortex*, *50*, 19–31.

Iacoboni, M. (2009). Imitation, empathy, and mirror neurons. *Annual Review of Psychology*, *60*, 653–70.

Kim, D-K., Lee, K-M., Kim, J., Whang M-C., & Kang, S. W. (2013). Dynamic correlations between heart and brain rhythm during Autogenic meditation. *Frontiers in Human Neuroscience*, *7*(414), 1–8.

Kurzban, R., & Aktipis, A. (2007). Modularity and the social mind: Are psychologists too selfish? *Personality and Social Psychology Review, 11*(2), 131–149.

Lazzari, C., Masiello, I., & Shoka, A. (2016). Improving team's self-awareness of stress-related events during Interprofessional Teamwork (IPT) in mental health. Identifying tools to reinforce the mind-brain education into psychiatric wards. *Proceedings of the Royal College of Psychiatrists International Congress*, 27–30 June 2016, London [in press].

Maxwell, B., & Racine, E. (2012). The ethics of neuroeducation: Research, practice and policy. *Neuroethics*, *5*, 101–103.

Miller, B. L., & Cummings, J. L. (Eds.) (2007). *The human rontal lobes: Functions and disorders* (2nd ed.). New York: The Guilford Press.

National Organization for Disorders of the Corpus Callosum (2016). Corpus callosum disorders. Retrieved from http://nodcc.org/.

Naumann, R. K., et al. (2015). The reptilian brain. *Current Biology*, *25*(8); R317–321.

Ringleb, A. H., & Rock, D. (2008). The emerging field of NeuroLeadership. *NeuroLeadership Journal*, *1*, 1–17.

Ritz, K., van Buchem, M. A., & Daemen, M. J. (2013). The heart-brain connection: Mechanistic insights and models. *Neth. Heart J. 21*, 55–57.

Rizzolatti, G., & Craighero, L. (2004). The mirror-neuron system. *Annu. Rev. Neurosci. 27*, 169–92.

Rochat, P., & Ferreira, P. (2008). Homo Negotiatus: Ontogeny of the unique ways humans own, share and reciprocate. In: Itakura, S., & Fujita, K. (Eds.). *Origins of the social mind: Evolutionary and developmental views.* Tokyo: Springer.

Rowe, A. D., Bullock, P. R., Polkey C. E., & Morris, R. G. (2001). Theory of mind impairments and their relationship to executive functioning following frontal lobe excisions. *Brain*, *124*, 600–616.

Sanders, R. (2014). Chronic stress primes brain for mental illness. The Regents of the University of California. Retrieved from http://www.universityofcalifornia.edu/news/chronic-stress-primes-brain-mental-illness.

Schnelle, H. (2010). *Language in the brain*. Cambridge: Cambridge University Press.

Slachevsky, A., & Dubois, B. (2004). Frontal assessment battery and differential diagnosis of frontotemporal dementia and Alzheimer diseases. *Archives of Neurology*, *61*(7), 1104–1107.

Stevens, C. (1998). Realism and Kelly's pragmatic constructivism. *Journal of Constructivist Psychology*, *11*(4), 283–308.

Taylor, K. J., Henson, R. N. A., & Graham, K. (2007). Recognition memory for faces and scenes in amnesia: Dissociable roles of medial temporal lobe structures. *Neuropsychologia*, *45*(11), 2428–2438.

Tsolaki, M., Eleftheriou, M., & Karavida, N. (2009). Alzheimer's dementia and post-traumatic stress disorder differences and similarities in neuroimaging. *Hell. J. Nucl. Med.* *12*(1), 41–6.

Vygotsky. L. (1978). *Mind in society: The development of higher psychological processes*. Cambridge, MA: Harvard University Press.

Waldman, D. A., Balthazard, P. A., & Peterson, S. J. (2011). Social cognitive neuroscience and leadership. *The Leadership Quarterly, 22*, 1092–1106.

Wertsch, J. V. (1985). *Vygotsky and the social formation of mind.* Cambridge, MA: Harvard University Press.

In: Communication Skills
Editor: Bridget L. Wright

ISBN: 978-1-63485-565-5

Chapter 4

DECISION-MAKING MODELS IN PATIENTS WITH DEPRESSION: A REVIEW OF HOW AND WHO SHOULD DECIDE

Hugo Sérgio Almeida[1,2]
and Margarida Figueiredo-Braga[1,3,*]

[1]Medical Psychology Unit,
Department of Clinical Neurosciences and Mental Health
Faculty of Medicine, University of Porto
[2]Hospital Magalhães Lemos E.P.E. Porto, Portugal
[3]I3S Instituto de Investigação e Inovação em Saúde

ABSTRACT

The clinical decision process is central to the patient-physician relationship. The paternalistic approach, once the preferential model of medical practice is now under severe criticism. Clinicians find themselves trying to find alternative models where the physician is not a sole source of information as in an Informed Decision Model, nor an agent to interpret the will and decide by the patient as in a Doctor-as-Agent Model. The Shared-Decision Model is in line with this endeavor, inviting the patient and physician to be co-responsible with the information exchange and treatment plan.

* Corresponding author: Al Prof Hernâni Monteiro, 4200-391 Porto, Email:mmfb@med.up.pt.

This model, based on strong communication ability, shows particular interest in the decisions that are sensitive to personal preferences and entail some degree of uncertainty – as the majority of the decisions made in the psychiatric field. Furthermore depression is thought to place patient's capability to decide at risk. The research shows however that patients with depression still want to participate in the clinical decisions, and reports a positive impact of using this model on the compliance with the therapeutic plan, in a decreased need of hospitalization and in better knowledge of the illness and higher satisfaction with health services. Shared-decision appears to be of additional interest, once it promotes the sense of autonomy and self-efficacy, decreasing feelings of helplessness and hopelessness associated with depressive state.

We performed a review of the models of decision making and its application to psychiatric patients. The reviewed literature permited to uncover the model characteristics more suitable to application in depressed patients and their physicians in the decision process. When dealing with patients with depression, sharing technical knowledge and information and the joined participation in the process of decision seems to be welcomed, and even desired. Results highlight the influence of a Shared-Decision Model on patient's satisfaction and compliance with treatment.

Keywords: decision-making, depression

INTRODUCTION

The patient-physician interaction is an essential component of medical practice. Central to this interaction is the communication between both and the relationship established. Patients came into clinical settings commonly seeking help, either searching for information or care, mostly in the search for a solution to their problem. However, the process of finding the right treatment and the answer for this endeavors is not straightforward and is largely dependent on the patient, the physician and the clinical situation.

Several decision-making processes have been described: from a paternalistic approach, built over an authoritarian view of the patient-physician relationship, to more contemporary models of shared decision-making, where a joint and co-responsible decision is aimed. The research on the decision making process, and its goals, has been done in parallel to the evolution of models of patient-physician relationship, highlighting how both influence and enable each other.

Physicians were historically seen as the embodiment of wisdom, alike ancient priests with almost divine powers. The ancient religious leaders helped the populations by translating god's laws. Every ail, health-related or otherwise, was seen as a fault, and for each fault there was an atonement in order. Dealing with eternal and unchanging laws, there was no place for negotiation between the sinful and the deity, just submission and expiation. With the dawn of Positivism, illnesses were no longer seen as punishments. The disease state became 'notisfault'[1] and so medicine began to brew new explanations and causality inferences between organic derangements and disease. This time, the knowledge of the physician did not came from the heavens, but was funded on scientific knowledge. However, still as hermeneutic and inaccessible for the layman as before. This is the relationship that Parson described in the 1950's, an interaction where the patient was committed to the passivity of the '*sick role*'. Parson [1] describes a helpless patient, whose technical incompetence hinders any chance of extricating out of illness by his own effort. In this paradigm, the physician is responsible for the welfare of patient, in line with a Paternalistic Model of decision-making. However this model imposes a considerable burden to physicians in conditions which are known to be uncontrollable or with a high degree of uncertainty.

Evidence-Based Medicine and Patient-Centered Care

Contemporary clinical practice is strongly influenced by empirical science, used as an explicit basis for making judgements about the provision of clinical care [2]. This model assumes that whatever treatment shown to be the most effective is the '*rational' choice to implement, and 'if an informed patient with expressed desire to get well chooses a different treatment this choice must be the result of wither unusual or irrational thinking* '[3]. Taken to extreme, evidence-based decision-making has been associated with rational decision-making, in which choices made by patients which deviate from the scientific evidence are labelled as irrational, from which the patient must be protected.

With the proposal of the biopsychosocial model of illness, which also emphasized the importance of psychosocial factors in the course of illness, the patient's experience of illness acquired a central role in decision-making [4]. The ilness centered-care paradigm was replaced by the patient-centered medicine, dethroning the scientific perspective and moving the patient from the periphery to the center of medical decision making [5]. Patient-centered care withdraw health care from the exclusive focus on symptoms and physiological outcomes, taking into account that patients often value functional outcomes and quality of life higher than control of illness. This challenges a science-based paradigm, assuming that the clients are the best judges of their own needs.

Formerly incompatible with either a shared or an informed model of clinical decision-making, the evidence-based approach is being redefined, considering that the scientific information is not exclusively advantageous to find a treatment option, but rather to help create more informed patients and enhance patient choice [6]. Intermingled with the principles of patient-centeredness, evidence-based medicine now assumes that client preferences, expressed as informed choices, outweigh scientific evidence [4].

Models of Patient-Physician Relationship

Medical treatments have become increasingly technologically complex and there is expected that they are justified by scientific evidence. However, taking into account the limitations of empirical health research, the patient-physician relationship has become increasingly valuable [7]. Contemporary with Parson, Szasz and Hollander [8] described three basic models of doctor-patient relationship, which translate into different approaches to treatmen t[8] – Table 1. The first model assumes that in some instances it might not be possible for the patient to participate in the relationship and the physician acquires an authoritarian posture - the Activity-Passivity Model. Conceptually, there is no interaction between patient and physician, since he is unable to contribute. Nowadays, with the increasing use of advance directives, this model may no longer be acceptable (even) in emergency situations.

The other two models assume that an interaction is established, both participants are 'active' in the sense that they contribute to what ensues from the relationship. However patient and physician's functions differ: in the Guidance-Cooperation Model the main difference pertains to power, and to its actual or potential use – the patient is expected to 'look up to' and to 'obey' his doctor; in the Mutual Participation Model, the power is divided and the participants are mutually interdependent, engaging in an interaction satisfying for both.

Table 1. Models of Physician-Patient Relationship and its' concepts of "Treatment"/"Therapeutic Result"

Model	*Physician's/ Patient's Role*	*Clinical Application of Model*	*Meaning of "Treatment"*	*Meaning of "Therapeutic Result"*
Activity-Passivity	Does something to patient/Recipient (inert or unresponsive)	1. Treatment of the unconscious patient; 2. Major surgical operation under general anesthesia	Whatever the physician does; the actual procedures which he employs	Alteration in the structure and/or function of the patient's body (or behavior, as determined by the physician); the patient's judgment does not enter into the evaluation or results
Guidance-Cooperation	Tells patient what to do/Cooperator (obeys)	Most of general medicine and the post-operative care of surgical patients		Patient's judgement is not irrelevant; success of therapy is still the physician's private decision; if patient agrees, he is a good patient, but if he disagrees he is bad or 'uncooperative'
Mutual Participation	Helps patient to help himself/Participant in 'partnership (uses expert help)	The treatment of patients with certain chronic diseases or permanent structural defects	An abstraction of one aspect of the relationship, embodying the activities of both participants; "treatment" does not take place unless both participants orient themselves to the task ahead	Evaluation of the result will depend on both the physician's and the patient's judgments and is further complicated by the fact that these may change in the very process of treatment

(Adapted from "*A contribution to the philosophy of medicine; the basic models of the doctor-patient relationship.*", Szasz, T. S. and M. H. Hollender (1956). AMA Arch Intern Med 97(5): 585-592.)

This last model is highly developed and pointed as ideal when dealing with chronic diseases, where the patient's experience provides reliable and important clues for therapy. Moreover, the treatment program is carried out by the patient, so that the *'physician helps the patient to help himself'[8]*. The Mutual Participation Model requires a complex psychological and social organization of both participants, and according to Szasz and Hollander, *'is rarely appropriate for children or for those persons who are mentally deficient, very poorly educated, or profoundly immature'[8].*

Those authors did not consider that patient's participation might extend to involvement in treatment decisions, neither that he could ever assume a dominant role in decision-making. Latter Freidson argued that the patient's status may be equal to, or even higher than that of the doctor – as in private practice. However, neither predicted consumer sovereignty in publicly financed health services [9].

Compliance (vs) Concordance Paradigms

Compliance is the degree a patient's behavior corresponds to the physician's prescription [10] and implies obedience to his authority [11], this definition highlights the power imbalance in the patient-physician relationship, hallmark of paternalistic models of medical practice, emphasizing pejorative obedience for the patient. It focuses more on behavior and less in the attitudes toward medication, failing to capture *'the dynamic complexity of autonomous patients, who must navigate decisional conflicts in learning to manage disorders over the course of decades'[5].*

This paradigm has been criticized for being too simplistic to address the complex decision-making processes that are required to discover the optimal use of medication. It devaluates the patient's role in health care decisions [5], blaming those who do not follow medical advice [12]. It assumes furthermore that the patient possess adequate information on the condition being treated and its treatment, has access to medication and the ability to take it as instructed, which is not always the case. Research that analyzed compliance from the patient's perspective found that the main reason why people choose not to follow physician's prescriptions concerned the drugs themselves [13]. Others were: as a way of expressing their attempts to cope with their disease, as a reaction to the way they were treated by physicians, or as a way of fighting the system by breaking its symbolic rules [12].

The more neutral concept of adherence aimed to surpass the concept of compliance, hoping that the term would not reflect the same degree of coercion [11]. Adherence definition according the World Health Organization is *'the degree to which the person's behavior corresponds with the agreed recommendations from a health care provider'*. Although it implies a more collaborative perspective by integrating the physician's medical opinion and the patient's lifestyle, values and preferences, the underlying paternalism remained, and a new model of concordance was proposed.

Concordance refers to *'anticipated outcome of the consultation between doctors and patients about medicine taking, if both parties can be encouraged to work together as partners'*. It differs from the previous concepts focusing on the consultation process rather than on a specific patient behavior, and has an underlying ethos of shared approach to decision-making [13, 14]. It advocates a sharing of power in the patient-physician relationship, ensuring they have enough information to participate in making decisions about treatment and supporting them with any problems they might have. Stevenson [15] defines three necessary elements for the concordance practice: the evidence that patients share their beliefs, experiences and preferences, that physicians question about health care preferences and constraints on adherence and that a balanced discussion takes place between health care practitioners and patients. "It is a process, which entertains patients' views on medication taking, and acknowledges that patients' views have to be respected even if they make choices, which appear to be in conflict with the clinician's views [16].

For this to be possible, doctors need to recognize patients' decision-making abilities, to try to understand patients' needs and constraints, and work with patients in the development of treatment regimens [12] - beyond a compliance paradigm, towards a therapeutic alliance – in line with share decision-making.

MODELS OF CLINICAL DECISION-MAKING

Increasing relevance is being attributed to the process of medical decision in clinical practice, which draws important characteristics from the interaction established. Several models of decision making have been identified, varying in the roles assumed by the patient and the physician, the relative sharing of information and the decision-making power.

Different models of treatment decision-making may be more or less appropriate, or feasible, in specific contexts (eg. emergency setting, long-term monitoring of medication in the treatment of chronic disorders, palliative care).

The health-related decision-making process is composed of two steps. The first one involves the evaluation of scientific evidence requiring analytic skills with the prospect that an agreement can be reached [17]. The second step comprises the subjective evaluation of facts, integrating personal values and inclinations. In a patient-centered paradigm, this appraisal should draw from the patient's preferences and be reflected into a meaningful decision. There are no correct answers, nor an obligation that an agreement is reached. The most prominent models of treatment decision-making are the Paternalistic, Informed and Shared-decision Models – Table 2.

1. Paternalistic Model of Decision-Making

Sometimes called parental, or priestly model, it derives from the early conceptualization of the 'sick role'. The physician is depicted as a guardian of the patient's best interest, without the need to elicit the latter's preferences. Submissiveness to professional authority is based on several assumptions [6]:

1. It assumes that a single best treatment exists, and that there are objective criteria for determining what that is;
2. Physicians know the best treatment available and consistently apply this knowledge when selecting treatments;
3. Physicians are in the best position to evaluate the tradeoffs between different treatment and therefore to make the treatment decision;
4. Physicians have a legitimate investment in each treatment decision, because of their professional concern for the welfare of their patients.

According to this model the patient assumes a passive role, in an encounter dominated by the physician, who uses his skills to diagnose and recommend test and treatments. If any, the patient involvement is limited to providing consent to these recommendations, thankful for the decisions made by the physician even if he would not agree to them at the time [12]. Differences in education, income and gender also contribute to this power disparity.

With the increasing number of illnesses for which no best treatment existed, the decisional context evolved to considerer different treatments with different types of tradeoffs between benefits and risks. The widespread variations in clinical practice underlined the changeable scientific basis of much medical care and heightened the awareness that doctor's values and beliefs influence clinical decisions [9]. Since the patient rather than the physician has to live with the consequences of the decisions, the assumption that the physician is in the best position to evaluate and weigh advantages and disadvantages was increasingly challenged [6]. The objectivity of the professionals has also been questioned given that several factors can cloud their objective judgement [7].

This model has been considered inappropriate for many current treatment decision-making contexts, and is presently limited to emergency situations, where the patient is not able to participate in the decision-making interaction, and there are no advance directives, or in the presence of incompetent patient without a guardian (e.g., under-aged people, some mentally ill patients).

The instrumental model represents the extreme version of the paternalistic approach to clinical decision making. It rests on an abusive disregard to the patient's values and well-being, such as disrespectful or unethical human experimentation. According to this model the physician acts on behalf of a goal independent of the patient, such as the good of society or the progress of scientific knowledge [16].

The logical next step appeared to be the patient empowerment in treatment decisions. Advocates of patient-centered care invoked two main arguments for increasing patient decisional-power [7]: a philosophical argument – the ethical principle of autonomy; and an economic argument – a free market concept where more consumer choice may increase standards through competition.

2. Informed Models of Decision-Making

Several models were developed in reaction to the paternalistic model. The Informed Models of Decision Making emerged from the recognition of informational asymmetry between patient and physician – technical knowledge resided in one party of the interaction, while personal preferences reside in the other These models postulate that both types of information need to be combined in the provision of effective care [18].

Informed Decision-Making Model

This model emphasizes patient sovereignty and patients' rights to make independent, autonomous choices. It embodies the adoption of business terms for medicine, as when physicians are described as health-care providers and patients as consumers [19]. This consumer oriented model, also called scientific or engineering model, rests on two assumptions [6]:

1. Patients possession of current scientific information on treatment enables them to make the best decision for themselves;

2. Physicians should not be involved in the decision-making process, since their interests and motivations may be different from the patients'.

The role of the physician is limited to information exchange, communicating the needed technical or scientific knowledge to the patient. This is seen as an enabling strategy, reducing the asymmetry in the clinical relationship by increasing the patient's knowledge. Patients should therefore be able to make decisions that reflect both their preferences and the best scientific knowledge available, no longer needing to share the treatment decision-making process.

This model also assumes a 'rational actor model' of information transfer, which assumes that the evidence-based information provided is fully understood as stated. Scientific evidence in the form of probability statements is transferred to the patient, who is perceived as a passive and empty vessel. It leaves no active role for the patient to interpret the scientific information or to try to make it personally meaningful [20].

The informative physician lacks a caring approach that requires understanding of the patient values, and his proscribed from giving recommendation for fear of imposing his will on the patient and thereby competing for the decision-making control that has been given to him [3]. It does not consider that an informed patient may still prefer not to lead the treatment decision-making process, ignoring that they are often uncertain and have 'second order desires', that is, the capacity to reflect on their wishes and to revise their own desires and preferences [3].

For these reasons this model is now being criticized, justified only where there is a one-time physician-patient interaction without an ongoing relationship in which the patient's values can be elucidated.

Interpretive Model

In the Interpretive Model [21] the role of the physician remains an informative one, however, he also helps to elucidate the patient's values and what he actually wants. It places the elucidation of values in the context of the patient's medical condition at the center of the physician-patient interaction. The physician informs and helps the patient to understand and use these values in the medical situation, leaving to him the ultimate decision.

The physician acts as a counselor, whose obligations include those enumerated in the informative model but also require engaging the patient in a joint process of self-understanding leading to autonomy.

Deliberate Model

According to this decision-making decision process [21] the physician acts as a teacher or friend, engaging the patient in a dialogue on what course of action would be best. The physician using no more than moral persuasion aims to suggest why certain health related values are more worthy and should be aspired to. Here, the conception of autonomy is moral self-development. The patient is empowered not to simply follow unexamined preferences or examined values, but to consider, through dialogue, alternative health related values, their worthiness and implications for treatment.

In this model the physician's values are relevant to patients. They inform their choice as a physician, who would not only help fit therapies to the patient's elucidated values, but also promote health-related principles. It embodies an ideal of a caring physician who integrates the information and relevant tenets to make a recommendation and, through discussion, attempts to persuade the patient to accept this recommendation.

Professional-as-Agent Model

Derived from economics, this model also resolves the asymmetry between the physician and patient, this time with information transfer from the patient to the physician. The patient gives information regarding self-knowledge, that the physician has no other way of knowing. The physician's role is one of an agent *'trying to choose what the patient would have chosen, had he been as well-informed as the professional'[18]*. The decision-making process is restricted to the physician, who is refrained from using his preferences – the only preferences that matter are those of the patient. The professional makes the decision, either assuming that they know, or having elicited the patient's preferences [2].

3. Collaborative Models of Decision-Making

The information sharing from the physician to the patient does not lead to a sharing of the decision-making process. This notion of two separate goals in the medical encounter – information sharing and decision-making sharing contributed to the emergence of a effective shared model of decision-making [18].

Shared-Decision Model

The Shared Decision-Making (SDM) model refers to a patient-physician communicational process, as part of the healthcare delivery, in which both participants collaborate to access information and enable health care decisions to be made [22]. Patient participation in the decision-making process regarding medical treatment encompasses a number of interests [2, 18]:

1. *Legal* - Widespread obligation of informed consent registry implies a minimum of shared decision-making;
2. *Ethical* - The emergence of consumer rights movement and the call for patients' autonomy, demands for a shared process that goes beyond informed consent to include broader principles of patient autonomy and control;
3. *Clinical* – With the shift in the nature of medical practice, from an acute to a more chronic care, caregivers often manage illnesses or combinations of illnesses rather than cure disease, which poses decisional challenges not solved by the sole use of empirical evidence.

This model seems to be of special interest when decisions are sensitive to personal preferences, such as facing uncertain or equivocal evidence of benefit [2]. In the management of chronic illness the patient necessarily is responsible for his own care [4]. To manage his condition, decision-making almost always involves different possibilities with different possible outcomes, and substantial uncertainty regarding impact on physical and psychological wellbeing [18].

Charles [18] sets four necessary criteria for classifying a physician-patient decision-making interaction as a Shared Decision-Making process: 1. *Quorum* - it must involve at least two active participants, comfortable with their level of participation; 2. *Information exchange* - both the physician and the patient share information; 3. *Joint deliberation* - both parties participate in the process of decision, expressing treatment preferences; and 4. *Decision* - a treatment decision is made upon the agreement of both parties.

To the active involvement of the two participants it is essential the respect for the patient's preferences. The physician must first elicit patient's preferences for participation in the decision-making process, give choices as to how this process will proceed and then respect patient's choices by behaving accordingly [18]. Research on patient's attitudes towards medical care revealed that patient vary in their preferred role in medical decision and they want to choose a physician with whom they can have a trusting relationship

[4]. Preferences for involvement may also fluctuate over time or depending on circumstances. Patients who express preferences for some form of shared decision-making do not necessarily act accordingly in the medical encounter. Therefore, physicians should regularly review patient's changing preferences for involvement, familiarizing themselves with the competing demands they experience at each decision-making stage [2] and consider situational factors surrounding the doctor-patient interaction [21]. Some patients prefer a passive role in the decision-making process [17]. In a study by Degner [23], 15% of participants believed that they had been forced to assume more responsibility for the decision than they were comfortable with. Those who prefer a more active role tend to be younger, more educated and healthier [9]. People with serious and chronic illnesses or older are less likely to prefer an active role in choosing treatments [5]. Older patients passivity may be explained by a cohort effect – they are cultural prone to see the doctor as a traditional power figure, a aging effect – they tend to rely more on the expertise of others and desire less responsibility in medical care, and/or a companion effect – they are more often accompanied by others participating in the decision-making process instead of the patient.

Limiting the conceptualization of SDM to a dyad may not reflect the current realities of clinical practice. The physician-patient interaction often involves more participants, with different patients, physicians, as well as relatives and friends. The range of interactional dynamics is automatically increased, and enables the formation of coalitions that will vary depending of the decisional context [18].

It is not always clear what type and amount of information patients want, or why they want it. Research suggests that physicians misestimate patient's preferences for information [24]. They are not so much interested in average outcomes for aggregate groups of patients as they are in knowing what this information means for themselves. Patients interpret information in order to make them personally meaningful [25]. They combine medical advice with information from other sources, ranging from health education campaigns and media articles to folklore and conversations with friends. All these sources are weighed in order to fit the patient's circumstances. Furthermore patients will use their own expertise about society and everyday life to decide how to use the medical information available [26].

Both patient and physician are required to bring their own expertise to the decision-process, sharing technical knowledge and personal information from both parties. Patients are increasingly literate in medical knowledge, and it is crucial for the physician to ascertain this health-related beliefs. Physicians' values are also important in that they enable the building of a professional opinion, not only based on raw empirical evidence, but on clinical and personal experience. This helps to bridge the empirical evidence base, which is established on population averages, with the unique concerns, values and life context of the individual patient [5]. On the other hand the value of information from the patient's perspective does not lie solely in its potential use as an aid to decision-making, but also as a psychological reassurance, reducing uncertainty at a time of great stress and vulnerability [27].

Agreement between physician and patient about the treatment decision is one possible outcome of a shared process; others include no decision or disagreement as to the preferred treatment. A shared decision does not mean that both parties are necessarily convinced that this is the best treatment possible, but rather endorse it as the treatment to implement - through mutual acceptance both parties share responsibility for the final decision [18].

With emphasis on interaction, based on the bidirectional exchange of information and joint process of deliberation, this model is likely to be more complex and time consuming than either the paternalistic or informed approaches, each of which require less interaction and consensus building [6]. SDM encourages a dialogue between patient and clinician to clarify overt and covert intervenient factors – socio-demographic and cultural, so as to reach treatment decisions which the patient will likely implement.

A number a benefits have been reported when shared decision-making is applied. From the clinical perspective, improvements in the therapeutic relationship as well as in a variety of health outcomes such as treatment adherence, satisfaction and biomedical outcomes were found. Patients who performed the decision-making role tend to be more satisfied and present a higher functional status. Surveys also demonstrate that near the totality of patient desire information on relevant healthcare problems and many want to participate in health care decisions. The application of a shared decision model also possesses economic advantages - as a consumer patient's control represents a mean of tying the healthcare industry into a form of market discipline. From a theoretical and ethical point of view shared decision-making is an end in itself due to the assumption that people with illnesses should determine what happens to their bodies and are best suited to make the decisions because only they can place personal values on the outcomes.

Concerns on possible disadvantages of offering patients a shared process of information exchange and decision have also been suggested [4, 9, 28-30]:

1. *Sense of overwhelming* – Choices can be debilitating for those who have difficulty with important decisions;
2. *Fear of decision regret/Increased sense of lost opportunities* – Patients may experience regret or reject options to spare themselves the possibility of regret;
3. *Difficulty in valuing outcomes* – Patients may be unable to anticipate how they will adapt to illness or react to treatment;
4. *Dissatisfaction with clinical realities* – The expectation of choice and decisional control may lead to dissatisfaction when expectations meet clinical realities;
5. *Discomfort with assuming unsought responsibility;*
6. *Nocebo effect* – Disclosing information about risks may increase the experience of adverse effects due to suggestibility;
7. *Impracticability* – Unfeasibility to provide information on the potential risks and benefits of all treatment options available;
8. *Utopic usage of resources* – Greater patient involvement in decision-making may lead to a greater demand for unnecessary, costly or harmful procedures which could undermine the equitable allocation of health resources;

There are situations in which shared decision making is not fully applicable, such as in emergency situations or in situations in which there is a decisional incapacity. In these situations, advance directives can help to protect the patient autonomy and provide practitioners with a guide to making treatment decisions that are conducted by the clients' preference and values – a method consistent with client-centered care and SDM [5].

Several interventions to improve patient's decisional capacities have been suggested, either from the physicians (e.g., improvement of clinicians skills [18]) or from the patients perspective (e.g., patient decision aids [2, 6, 18], communication skills programs [18, 31], individual preparation of patients).

DECISION-MAKING IN PSYCHIATRY

Since 1970s, the process of negotiating a treatment approach, with the attainment of a mutually acceptable option between the patient and the physician, has been discussed in psychiatry. The roles played and the imbalance of power between physicians and patients, have been questioned with the rising of cultural and professional movements such as the anti-psychiatry movement, consumer-led services, the alternative treatment movement and the critical psychiatry networks [7]. The evolving policy of informed consent including patient's values define physicians interventions aiming to enhance patient's control over their options, treatment, health and lives [32]. The participation of patients in medical decisions affecting their treatment is increasingly being advocated in the field of mental health [33]. This desire and the need to frame medication within the context of the client's desires, life goals and history, brought the concept of therapeutic alliance to the frontline of psychiatric practice [5]. This alliance implies a collaborative approach, based on co-responsibility and trust hopefully translating into better clinical and personal outcomes, with careful consideration of both consumer and provider perspectives.

Most studies show that people with mental illnesses are interested in being involved in the management of their conditions, and welcome opportunities to be informed and share the process of decision-making [2, 6, 34]. Patients consistently report positive attitudes towards shared-decision making [32, 35, 36], with levels of interest higher than those experienced [6, 37, 38, 39]; and similar [36] or higher [33, 38] than patients with somatic diseases.

The patient's desire to be informed about his mental condition and treatment has been shown to be higher than the desire to participate in decision-making [33, 40, 41]. They seek information about their illness, welcome scientific evidence and like to be kept up-to-date about illness and treatment as well as other supports within the mental health system [42]. This information is frequently not volunteered by physicians [39] or other health professionals, forcing patient to be proactive in obtaining information, either in the consultation, or with other professionals, family, social contacts, and/or digital resources. Similar levels of desire for information were found in all ages [43]. However the decision aid material created for general health does not translate perfectly to mental health. The power differential, coupled with providers' ability to use legal means to override consumer preferences, creates a different dynamic in psychiatric practice [44]. There is moreover a lack of instructions to providers on the use of such aids, and the limited technical assistance makes them difficult to implement.

Decisional conflict in psychiatric patients may be explained by stigma, symptom suppression, and delayed onset of consequences due to discontinuation of medicine. This highlights the need for support resolving the ambivalence regarding the use of psychiatric medications or other therapeutic tools [5].

Patients have a strong desire to be involved in decisions about their medications [38], but fear taking full control or responsibility over the decision taken or the treatment to follow [33, 36]. They wish a collaborative approach [45], rather than an informative or paternalistic model. A tendency to prefer a lesser role in the decision-making process was exclusively found when more severe clinical pictures were present [45].

Preferences appear to vary in relation to the type of decision being made. Patients prefer to assume a collaborative role when facing psychiatric medications, an autonomous role for decisions related to psychosocial interventions, and a passive role with their primary care provider [38, 43]. Psychiatrists, on the other hand consider psychosocial and lifestyle issues to be more suitable for shared decision-making than medical or legal decisions [46].

Differences in participation preferences across different psychiatric conditions are negligible [36] and demographic or situational variables explain less than 20% of the variability in decision-making preferences [47]. Research reports higher desire to participate in decisions in patients with:

1. *Experience of involuntary treatment [33]*
   In mental health some patients may be forced to treatment but even in those treated involuntarily, some degree of autonomous choice is possible. This partial inclusion in treatment decisions may improve their attitude toward treatment and thus enhance compliance.
2. *Negative attitudes toward treatment [33]*
   Patients unsatisfied with treatment, namely those with less insight into the necessity of treatment [37], expectation of side effects or uncertain of treatment benefits [32], are more likely to non-adherent. When dealing with patients with poor insight and negative drug attitudes, psychiatrists tend to use authoritative decision-making styles despite the patient desire to participate [37].
3. *Younger age [40, 45]*
   Studies report higher desire to participate in younger patients or in those with greater experience of living with illness. Others suggest that older adults are more likely to experience a passive role in psychiatry medication decisions [43].
4. *Female gender [36]*
5. *Higher education [36]*

Regarding mental health problems SDM is being practiced at the level of information exchange in both psychiatric and primary care setting [48]. Observational studies accurately assessing the SDM process in mental health consultations have found that the majority of professionals do not objectively favor involving the patient in the decision-making process [49-53]. Physicians report higher levels of patient's participation than those experienced by the patient, who state little meaningful input into major decisions, especially about medications [37, 44].

This discrepancy underscores the importance of explicitly inquiring the patient's preference in the decision-making process. Occasionally professionals, even if interested in a SDM process, resist directly asking patients about their preferences for involvement in decision-making [49] and describe to intuitively feel if the patient is able and interested in participating. Some investigators explain this behavior as a defensive routine, managing the environment unilaterally and controlling the task [49]. When patients initiate discussion about treatment options, however, physicians respond with greater patient involvement [52].

Taking into account patient preferences in treatment planning and delivery has been associated with several positive outcomes [44, 54] namely greater knowledge, satisfaction with treatment, feelings of being helped, involvement and activation of decision-making and improvement of treatment adherence with lower need for re-hospitalization [55-57].

Nonadherence to treatment in mental health is high and the lowest adherence rates are found in chronic conditions, when treatment is prophylactic or suppressive or the consequences of stopping treatment are delayed [58, 59]. Decisions regarding treatment are moreover influence by patient's expectations, attributions and believes, as exemplified below:

1. The patient may perceive treatment as "worse" than the disorder [5, 39, 60], either by the presence of intolerable side effects or by the experience of a transformation of self into a "drugged me" or a "not-me"
2. Using medication is seen as not worth the discrimination and social rejection associated [13, 39, 61, 62]
3. Treatment is an unwanted reminder of illness [63]
4. There is no need for treatment because they are not certain of being actually ill [13, 63]

5. Medications is needed to deal exclusively with specific symptoms, or when the symptoms are present and experienced as distressing.
6. It is best not to use medications because it is ineffective [64]

The concept of shared-decision making is also relevant to health decisions such as lifestyle modifications. Given the high morbidity and mortality of psychiatric populations, and the deleterious effects of psychiatric medication, promoting healthy lifestyles can have a major impact [64]. The model allows the physician to help the patient to identify personal resources as self-initiated, non-pharmaceutical self-care activities that serve to decrease symptoms, avoid undesirable outcomes such as hospitalization, and improve mood, thoughts, behaviors and wellbeing [60]. Nevertheless patients do not routinely disclose their personal resources and coping mechanisms to physicians and physicians do not routinely inquire about them. These strategies optimize the process of managing illness and promote health [45]. Physicians should learn to monitor their use.

The Recovery Model applied to mental health emphasizes and supports each individual's potential for recovery, seen as a personal journey that involves choice, self-determination, and empowerment [2]. Mastering a sense of self-efficacy that fostered accomplishment, control, and improvement in one's life have been found to be essential to recovery in psychiatric disorders [65]. A mismatch between treatment priorities and needs of patients with serious and persistent mental illness results in a fail to provide integration in the community [66]. Conversely, patient's participation in the decision-making process contribute to his autonomy and reinforce self-confidence.

Research reports diverse, and sometimes contradictory results regarding outcomes associated with SDM. There is a tendency to consider the shared approach to decision making as beneficial regarding commitment to therapy [67, 68], but no clear effects on clinical outcomes have been fond [7, 67, 69-71]. Chan and Mak described in 2012 four ways in which share decision-making could play a role in promoting aspects of mental health recovery [22]:

1. In the personal involvement and intimate commitment to the process of illness management and recovery. A recovery-oriented dialogue links the patients lived experience to their own concepts and understanding of recovery, and with this a new personal vision can be created, constituting a self-transformation of the patient. A recovery-oriented care for people with severe mental illness implies that the person in treatment should have the greatest role possible in

collaborating with the provider to define the goals of treatment and plan for ways to reach these goals [72].

2. Empowerment and reinforcement of a sense of self-direction. Patients with severe psychiatric symptoms seem to be less empowered and experience diminished self-confidence, which was not found to be correlated with global functioning. Instead, those with larger social support network reported more self-orientation to empowerment [73], including self-esteem and efficacy, community confidence and optimism. Greater self-orientation was associated with better quality of life, fewer symptoms and better social support [73]. The impact of empowerment on the community is manifested by the patients' desire to change his stigmatizing community. Patients believe they have some power within society, are interested in affecting change, and wish to promote community action [73].
3. Improvement of patient-physician relationship, by reducing the informational and decision-making asymmetry. Therapeutic relationship is an independent predictor of treatment outcome, a mediating factor that captures significant variance in the outcome of treatment interventions such as pharmacological therapies, and an outcome *per se* [74]. Schizophrenic patients who formed good therapeutic alliances with their therapists, for example, where found to be significantly more likely to remain in therapy, comply with the prescribed medication regimens, and achieve better outcomes with less medication [75].
4. Assurance of the selection and implementation of a consumer-desired plan.

Implementing SDM in psychiatric settings presents several difficulties. Fragmented services, learned helplessness, prejudice, discrimination and the fear of coercive consequences can challenge psychiatric patient's ability to actively and fully engage in shared decision-making [44]. Research shows, however, that those with severe mental health illness are able to participate in decision-making [48, 76], and that legal definitions of impaired competency to make health decisions affect only a minority of people diagnosed with mental disorders namely those with dementia or learning disabilities [2].

Among other problems patients commonly mention time restrictions as a barrier against SDM behaviors. It takes time to share information and preferences for treatments and to negotiate a course of action, as indicated by the finding that greater SDM behaviors are associated with longer visit duration [39, 49, 52, 77]. For instance discussion of health behaviors using SDM in the negotiation of behavior change is feasible in a 15- to 20-minute visit [50]. Consultation setting and organizational characteristics was also found to influence SDM behaviors. Physicians working in a health maintenance organization practice made fewer attempts to involve patients in the decision process [52], constrained by organizational factors such as formularies and treatment guidelines.

Culturally influenced attitudes and customs may represent facilitators or barriers to patient participation. Discrepancies in the ethnic, racial, cultural or social background of physicians and patients where described as obstacles to gather information regarding preferences and sharing decision-making processes [77].

Communication skills as the use of language that patients could understand, ability to negotiate and provide information where mentioned by physicians as facilitating a more co-operative relationship and simplify the decision-making task [39].

Shared decision-making is not suitable to all mental health situations. Autonomy of the patient should prevail in elective procedures or when treatment decisions are more controversial. However, in emergency and life-threatening situations, some authors consider that the paternalistic approach may still be desirable [7]. Due to acute and severe illness, an individual may be withdrawn from the decision process because of his inability to consciously participate. However, following improvement in their health status, he may be able to make a choice regarding continuing therapy. This change in ability should be accompanied by a change in the decision-making model used, supported by the physicians [39]. Even in situations where patient's decision-making capacity may be affected by the pathology, Psychiatric Advance Directives, where the person sets out their wishes beforehand, could be used[78]. These documents allow patients with severe and chronic mental illnesses to notify their treatment preferences for future crisis or relapses and to appoint a surrogate decision-maker for a period of incompetence. A recent review of the effects of advance treatment directives for people with severe mental illnesses provided little evidence on the benefits of these directives. Their completion rates remain very low [79] although well-suited for conveying patients' preferences congruently with patient-centered care.

Decision-Making in Patients with Depression

Van Grieken and coworkers [80] identified several characteristics of psychiatric treatment negatively influencing recovery, engagement in treatment and clinical outcome in major depressive disorder (MDD):

1. Lack of clarity and consensus regarding the nature of the disorder and its treatment between patients and clinicians;
2. Precarious relationship with the clinician;
3. Unavailability of mental healthcare when needed;
4. Insufficient involvement of significant others.

All these characteristics may impinge shared-decision, which is only recently been discussed in depressive care. The extension of shared decision making to the psychiatric context and in particular to depression reveals that most patients with depression are seeking information about their illness and treatment, and desire a collaborative involvement.

Preferences for involvement vary in different patients and within patients over time. They frequently revisit decisions, requiring ongoing decision support [81], especially during antidepressant therapy [82]. It is common for the same patient to experience both collaborative and paternalistic models in different decisional contexts. Preferences for involvement may not always fit the main models of involvement, requiring more flexible processes incorporating complex combinations. Older patients are more likely to accept a more traditional, dominant role for the physician, and report less confidence in discussing treatment options [47]. Less involvement is also experienced by inpatient in detoxification and forensic units [83], or whenever more difficult decisions have to be performed [84]. On the contrary, younger [83] patients and those with depression [35] demonstrate a greater level of interest for an active role in decision-making.

Patients with depression have frequently limited knowledge on the availability and efficacy of psychiatric treatments [85-87] and (moreover) convey to the clinical encounter various preconceived treatment preferences [88]. Raue and coworkers suggest that acknowledging patient's *a priori* treatment preferences may be conceptualized as a pre-shared decision-making strategy. A fully developed SDM intervention would determine the patient's preferences and also engage him/her in a dialogue about these preferences, review patient decision-aid materials, and conclude with a formulation satisfactory to both the patient and the clinician [88].

Previous experience with a treatment modality was found to be the strongest predictor of preference, with some contradictory results [89]. Preference for counseling therapies [71, 86, 90-96] or psychotherapy [62, 89, 97-105] is high, compared to medication. Individuals who believe that their depression has more serious consequences on their lives and attribute their depression to marital, family or interpersonal problems are prone to prefer psychotherapy [101]. Higher education is also related to psychotherapy preference. Depressed patients frequently attribute improved well-being to psychotherapy [102], but rarely to antidepressant medication, being less likely to believe that their underlying problems can be solved with just medication [89]. In clinical settings however most patients receive medication, meaning that less than 50% receive the therapy they prefer [86, 101].

On the other side, although a collaborative care model may improve the access to the preferred treatment, meeting a patient's preference appears not to affect symptom reduction or remission rates [71, 92, 99, 106].

The majority of patients report the need for more information in order to improve the decision-making process. Concerns about depression treatments including fears about the addictive and harmful properties of antidepressants, worries about taking "too many pills" and the stigma attached to taking psychotropic medication [62] are mainly discussed with the psychiatrist, but other sources of information (other professionals, social contacts or media) may be used as decision aids [81, 84]. Patients feel the need for basic information about illness and treatment options [76] drew on existing personal knowledge in order to be personally meaningful and accurate [83]. Low preferences for information are associated with higher depression scores and increasing age [107] with some patients declaring to feel unable to ask the information they need to be involved in the decision-making process [83]. Patients with all severity grades of depression are highly interested in information, but moderately interested in participating in decision-making [87].

Pharmacotherapy has become the main modality of depression treatment, but its efficacy is reduced by low patient adherence and premature discontinuation [108-110]. Low adherence is associated with unrealistic expectations [111], lack of treatment efficacy or unacceptable adverse effects [101], and discrepancy between symptom relief and cure [110]. The selection of the best antidepressant drug is difficult. There is a lack of evidence on their comparative effectiveness [112, 113], no perfect drug [114]; and clinicians struggle to delivery this information meaninfully while dealing with their own preferences [115-117].

In a study on the physicians perspective of the decision-making process [118], they reported to provide a description of the disorder and to mention the potential risks and benefits of medication, without discussing the potential outcomes of therapy. The most common topic was about the risks of taking medication, including side effects. The initial collaborative approach does not require exhaustive information to the patient, but requires a clear communication about [119]:

1. The chosen drug;
2. Treatment doses and time;
3. Time needed for the therapeutic response;
4. Potential side effects and ways to alleviate them;
5. Expected length of treatment;
6. General idea of drug mechanism and action.

Patients receiving this kind of information are more educated and have more positive initial beliefs about their medication. Consequently they are more likely to maintain follow up appointments and refer to be more satisfied with treatment. Aikens and colleagues propose specific educational messages to improve adherence during the first month of antidepressant therapy [120] taking into account the patient's beliefs about the disease and about medication, and tailoring the physician behavior to his preferences and expectations [121].

Information must be tailored according patient's age, education and literacy and the presence of cognitive impairment inherent to the disorder [88]. Physicians generally report to convey information orally and use fact-sheets from public or not-for-profit organizations. A recent article [117] reports that the use of depression decision aids improves the decision-making process, but no differences were detected in the evolution of depressive symptoms, remission rate or responsiveness to treatment.

Etiologic attributions of depressed patients were found to vary across cultural groups [62, 104, 122-126], and Vega et al. [127] emphasize the importance of communicating with depressed patients in their own language, using a participatory decision-making style intrinsic to the patient's culture, attending to culturally guaranteed expressions of depression. These explanatory models may assign milder illness attributions to depression and influence help-seeking choices, acceptance to proposed treatments and treatment preferences [125, 128].

As an example, religion beliefs can influence help-seeking and service utilization [129-131]. Correlations were found between religious involvement and major depressive disorder: lower prevalence among persons who use religious coping (attending religious services weekly) and higher prevalence in those who listen to religious radio programs [132]. Shared decision making interventions should support complementary and faith-based approaches as treatment adjuncts when appropriate and help patients articulate their beliefs about depression's etiology, severity and factors [88].

In primary care, first visits of patients with depressive symptoms showed a low rate of SDM behaviors [52]. These behaviors did not vary with the severity of the symptoms, but were influenced by the setting, patient-initiated requests for medication and physicians age [133]. This is consistent with the finding of lack of patient's involvement in treatment decisions in consultations about depression [53]. In contrast physicians report to employ a collaborative approach to the decision-making process, leaving the ultimate decision to the patient, unless they were being treated involuntarily [118]. Interestingly physicians relayed on their ability to gauge non-verbal cues rather than asking the patients explicitly how and if they wanted to be involved in SDM.

From the physician point of view several reasons were mentioned to abide for a collaborative approach to decision making in depression [118]: patient's involvement may be therapeutic itself, facilitates engagement and responsibility. Even though, they described several situations where they would not follow this model, possibly including caregivers in the decision-making process:

1. Severity of depressive symptoms and the associated decline in functioning;
2. Perceived risk levels, to self or others;
3. Perceived/own assumption of client preference of involvement;
4. Age or developmental stage of the client.

Concerns on decisional capacity are also raised in depression with some authors reporting a high use of maladaptive decision-making coping patterns [134] like decision avoidance and irrational decisions. An inverse correlation between severity of illness and confidence about decision-making was also found and the authors concluded that '*the greater the level of decisional conflict, the lower the level of confidence, the higher the level of irrational choice, and the more pessimistic and distorted was information processing*'.

Other authors on the contrary, found no association between depressive symptoms and the level of performance on the decision-making process [135].

Patients perceived a collaborative approach to decision making when physicians considered their opinion, talked with them about different treatment options and then mutually agreed on a decision [84]. Generally, according to observational studies, physicians tend to focus on the problem definition stage, failing to offer to the patient a variety of treatment options [53].

In depression it is common to involve more participants than the patient-physician dyad in decision-making. Caregivers and other relatives are often present in the consultation, particularly in the elderly. They have important supportive roles in line with the desired by the patient [83, 118, 136].

Potential negative outcomes of involving caregivers were cited by physicians, such as disagreements, critical or unhelpful comments or difficulties in establishing boundaries for clinicians not offering family therapy [118]. Research shows conflicting results regarding the influence of the involvement of caregivers in the presence of depressive symptoms [136]. Pressure from others may contribute to higher levels of decisional conflict. Family dynamics may be mostly powerful among particular ethnic groups [88, 104]. When disagreements with caregivers arose, physicians were reported to respond by involving caregivers earlier in the process, exploring and understanding the perspective of the caregiver, or restating the rationale or justification for their position [118].

It is claimed that SDM may directly alleviate key depressive symptoms, such as helplessness and hopelessness, indirectly improving clinical outcomes by increasing patient adherence [88]. While some studies show that this involvement has positive effects regarding treatment acceptance [86], adherence [137], clinical outcomes [138] and satisfaction with treatment [139, 140], others fail to show these benefits [71, 90].

When considering uniquely the patient treatment preference component of SDM a positive influence has been detected in treatment initiation [99] and adherence, but not in clinical outcomes [71, 92, 99, 106, 141, 142]. Patients who enact involvement roles consistent with their preferences report greater satisfaction or reduced depression than those with mismatches [133]. However, preference strength for assigned treatment, but not simply congruence, was associated with better treatment initiation and adherence [99]. Congruence of preferences per se with assigned treatment was related with treatment initiation, but not adherence. This findings suggest that when preferences lack intensity or are similarly intense, the most accessible treatment should be offered first. Alternatively, where patient treatment preferences are particularly strong, that option should be offered [99].

Reasons for the patient involvement included: engagement process, adherence to treatment, safety, autonomy and empowerment [83]. This involvement surpasses traditional treatment type decisions, including decisions about location of care and employment. Negative aspects of involving patients were also mentioned, such as disengagement from treatment, refusal of a treatment option that could offer some benefit and overwhelming of the patient when they were unwell [118].

Dealing with decision-making in depressive disorders implies considering specific difficulties namely the perception of the disorder including the stigma, the delay in seeking help and the absence of information given to patients about depression treatment options [84]. These specificities may represent barriers for a shared-decision-making approach, which may be grouped in four categories [83, 118]:

1. *Patient or caregiver related*: depressive symptoms, level of risk assigned to patient, poor engagement, preconceived perceptions (e.g., perception of paternalism and coerciveness), confidentiality, family conflict;
2. *Physician related*: lack of communication, breaks in trust, reluctance to disclose side-effects, disagreement between professionals, different styles and approaches to individual patients, disorganization, underestimation of patient's abilities;
3. *Service related*: time constrains, a aprioristic decisions, inpatient settings, accessibility;
4. *Broader*: stigma, lack of evidence, restriction of funding.

It has been suggested that this barriers can be overcome by explicitly offering involvement when making decisions about treatment, and involving the caregivers when appropriate [83]. Stigmatization may be avoided by treatment in general practice [91], but patients were aware of the limited treatment options available in this setting [84]. For older patients, for example, accessibility and stigma can be particularly troublesome, and they may be persuaded to use natural herbal remedies rather than evidence-based therapies, or misconstrue depressive symptoms as natural consequences of aging or medical illness, minimizing the need for treatment [143]. Older adults who met diagnostic criteria for mental disorders were less likely to perceive a need for mental health care, to receive specialty mental health care or counseling, or to receive referrals from primary care to mental health specialty care than young or middle-aged adults [144-146].

Time constrains are present in current medical system. Patients request substantially more time to communicate with their physician [102]. Time pressure has been considered a barrier to SDM; research in primary care settings regarding depression treatment found that the longer the consultation time, the higher scores on decision-sharing behaviors were reported [49]. However, these behaviors, while increasing patient participation and satisfaction, did not increased consultations time significantly [140].

Conversely some factors were already identified which contribute to facilitate SDM such as: adequate time, culture of the team, treating voluntary clients, having referral options, professional culture and a general shift in healthcare culture towards collaborative approaches and informed clients [118].

Conclusion

The patient-physician relationship is embodied with therapeutic actions. The communication between both and with the social network around becomes central to the process of cure. In this rich discussion between medical knowledge, its individualization to the patient's reality and the patient values, preferences and needs, there is a tendency for the patient to take the frontline.

Shared-decision appears to be the ideal commitment in the majority of clinical situations, even in most psychiatric settings. When dealing with patients with depression, sharing technical knowledge and information and the joined participation in the process of decision seems to be welcomed, and even desired. The consequent decision model promotes feelings of self-value and capacity, aspects withdrawn by the illness and valuable to the recovery.

This idealized collaboration poses new challenges to the physician in developing new strategies for interacting and new ways of navigating the relationship with the psychiatric patient, focused in understanding, towards a new and better care. In order to use a model of shared disease management, there are new habits and skills that need to be learnt. On the patient side, there is a necessity to promote autonomy and empower him with the necessary information to exercise it, training his ability to disclose preferences and tenets. On the physician side, there is a need to defy the paternalistic approach and help the patient to develop self-efficacy and exert more control. This means increased demands on the communication ability and deliberation skills of both intervenient. Only fulfilling this requirements, the proposed benefits of a shared relationship will become real and translate into measurable personal and clinical outcomes.

REFERENCES

[1] Parsons, T. The Situation Of Medical Practice. *The Social System*: Free Press, 1951. p. 296-322.

[2] Perestelo-Perez, L; Gonzalez-Lorenzo, M; Perez-Ramos, J; Rivero-Santana, A; Serrano-Aguilar, P. Patient involvement and shared decision-making in mental health care. *Curr Clin Pharmacol.*, 2011, 6(2), 83-90.

[3] Brock, DW; Wartman, SA. When competent patients make irrational choices. *The New England journal of medicine.*, 1990, 322(22), 1595-9.

[4] Adams, EL. Shared Decision-Making and Evidence-Based Practice., 2006.

[5] Deegan, PE; Drake, RE. Shared decision making and medication management in the recovery process. *Psychiatric services* (Washington, DC)., 2006, 57(11), 1636-9.

[6] Charles, C; Gafni A Fau - Whelan, T; Whelan, T. Decision-making in the physician-patient encounter: revisiting the shared treatment decision-making model., 1999(0277-9536 (Print)).

[7] Laugharne, R; Priebe, S. Trust, choice and power in mental health: a literature review. *Social psychiatry and psychiatric epidemiology.*, 2006, 41(11), 843-52.

[8] Szasz, TS; Hollender, MH. A contribution to the philosophy of medicine: the basic models of the doctor-patient relationship. *AMA archives of internal medicine.*, 1956, 97(5), 585-92.

[9] Coulter, A. Partnerships with patients: the pros and cons of shared clinical decision-making. *Journal of health services research & policy.*, 1997, 2(2), 112-21.

[10] Horne, R. Compliance, adherence, and concordance: implications for asthma treatment. *Chest.*, 2006, 130(1 Suppl), 65s-72s.

[11] Weiden, PJ; Rao, N. Teaching medication compliance to psychiatric residents: placing an orphan topic into a training curriculum. *Academic psychiatry: the journal of the American Association of Directors of Psychiatric Residency Training and the Association for Academic Psychiatry.*, 2005, 29(2), 203-10.

[12] Donovan, JL; Blake, DR. Patient non-compliance: deviance or reasoned decision-making? *Soc Sci Med.*, 1992, 34(5), 507-13.

[13] Pound, P; Britten, N; Morgan, M; Yardley, L; Pope, C; Daker-White, G; et al. Resisting medicines: a synthesis of qualitative studies of medicine taking. *Soc Sci Med.*, 2005, 61(1), 133-55.

[14] Marjorie Weiss, NB. Concordance: What is concordance? *The Pharmaceutical Journal.*, 2003.

[15] Stevenson, FA; Cox, K; Britten, N; Dundar, Y. A systematic review of the research on communication between patients and health care professionals about medicines: the consequences for concordance. *Health Expect.*, 2004, 7(3), 235-45.

[16] Chakrabarti, S. What's in a name? Compliance, adherence and concordance in chronic psychiatric disorders. *World Journal of Psychiatry.*, 2014, 4(2), 30-6.

[17] decision aoa., 1990.

[18] Charles, C; Gafni, A; Whelan, T. Shared decision-making in the medical encounter: what does it mean? (or it takes at least two to tango). *Soc Sci Med.*, 1997, 44(5), 681-92.

[19] Beisecker, AE. Aging and the desire for information and input in medical decisions: patient consumerism in medical encounters. *The Gerontologist.*, 1988, 28(3), 330-5.

[20] Charles, C. doing nothing is no choice charles., 1998.

[21] Emanuel, EJ; Emanuel, LL. Four models of the physician-patient relationship. *Jama.*, 1992, 267(16), 2221-6.

[22] Chan, KK; Mak, WW. Shared decision making in the recovery of people with schizophrenia: the role of metacognitive capacities in insight and pragmatic language use. *Clinical psychology review.*, 2012, 32(6), 535-44.

[23] Degner, LF; Kristjanson, LJ; Bowman, D; Sloan, JA; Carriere, KC; O'Neil, J; et al. Information needs and decisional preferences in women with breast cancer. *Jama.*, 1997, 277(18), 1485-92.

[24] Strull, WM; Lo, B; Charles, G. Do patients want to participate in medical decision making? *Jama.*, 1984, 252(21), 2990-4.

[25] Adelsward, V; Sachs, L. The meaning of 6.8: numeracy and normality in health information talks. *Soc Sci Med.*, 1996, 43(8), 1179-87.

[26] Turney, J. Public understanding of science. *Lancet* (London, England)., 1996, 347(9008), 1087-90.

[27] Mooney, G; Ryan, M. Agency in health care: getting beyond first principles. *Journal of health economics.*, 1993, 12(2), 125-35.

[28] Loomes, G; Sugden, R. Regret Theory: An Alternative Theory of Rational Choice Under Uncertainty. *The Economic Journal.*, 1982, 92(368), 805-24.

[29] Jansen, SJ; Kievit, J; Nooij, MA; Stiggelbout, AM. Stability of patients' preferences for chemotherapy: the impact of experience. *Medical decision making: an international journal of the Society for Medical Decision Making.*, 2001, 21(4), 295-306.

[30] Edelaar-Peeters, Y; Stiggelbout, AM. Anticipated adaptation or scale recalibration? *Health and Quality of Life Outcomes.*, 2013, 11, 171.

[31] Dowell, J; Jones, A; Snadden, D. Exploring medication use to seek concordance with 'non-adherent' patients: a qualitative study. *The British Journal of General Practice.*, 2002, 52(474), 24-32.

[32] Bunn, MH; O'Connor, AM; Tansey, MS; Jones, BD; Stinson, LE. Characteristics of clients with schizophrenia who express certainty or uncertainty about continuing treatment with depot neuroleptic medication. *Archives of psychiatric nursing.*, 1997, 11(5), 238-48.

[33] Hamann, J; Cohen, R; Leucht, S; Busch, R; Kissling, W. Do patients with schizophrenia wish to be involved in decisions about their medical treatment? *The American journal of psychiatry.*, 2005, 162(12), 2382-4.

[34] Deegan, PE; Rapp, C; Holter, M; Riefer, M. Best practices: a program to support shared decision making in an outpatient psychiatric medication clinic. *Psychiatric services* (Washington, DC)., 2008, 59(6), 603-5.

[35] Arora, NK; McHorney, CA. Patient preferences for medical decision making: who really wants to participate? *Medical care.*, 2000, 38(3), 335-41.

[36] Hamann, J; Neuner, B; Kasper, J; Vodermaier, A; Loh, A; Deinzer, A; et al. Participation preferences of patients with acute and chronic conditions. *Health Expect.*, 2007, 10(4), 358-63.

[37] Hamann, J; Kruse, J; Schmitz, FS; Kissling, W; Pajonk, FG. Patient participation in antipsychotic drug choice decisions. *Psychiatry research.*, 2010, 178(1), 63-7.

[38] Adams, JR; Drake, RE; Wolford, GL. Shared decision-making preferences of people with severe mental illness. *Psychiatric services* (Washington, DC)., 2007, 58(9), 1219-21.

[39] Smith, F; Francis, SA; Rowley, E. Group interviews with people taking long-term medication; comparing the perspectives of people with arthritis, respiratory disease and mental health problems. *International Journal of Pharmacy Practice.*, 2000, 8(2), 88-96.

[40] Ende, J; Kazis, L; Ash, A; Moskowitz, MA. Measuring patients' desire for autonomy: decision making and information-seeking preferences among medical patients. *Journal of general internal medicine.*, 1989, 4(1), 23-30.

[41] Nease, RF; Jr. Brooks, WB. Patient desire for information and decision making in health care decisions; the Autonomy Preference Index and the Health Opinion Survey. *Journal of general internal medicine.*, 1995, 10(11), 593-600.

[42] Tanenbaum, SJ. Consumer perspectives on information and other inputs to decision-making: implications for evidence-based practice. *Community mental health journal.*, 2008, 44(5), 331-5.

[43] O'Neal, EL; Adams, JR; McHugo, GJ; Van Citters, AD; Drake, RE; Bartels, SJ. Preferences of older and younger adults with serious mental illness for involvement in decision-making in medical and psychiatric settings. *The American journal of geriatric psychiatry: official journal of the American Association for Geriatric Psychiatry.*, 2008, 16(10), 826-33.

[44] Curtis, LC; Wells, SM; Penney, DJ; Ghose, SS; Mistler, LA; Mahone, IH; et al. Pushing the envelope; shared decision making in mental health. *Psychiatric rehabilitation journal.*, 2010, 34(1), 14-22.

[45] Hill, SA; Laugharne, R. Decision making and information seeking preferences among psychiatric patients. *Journal of Mental Health.*, 2006, 15(1), 75-84.

[46] Hamann, J; Mendel, R; Cohen, R; Heres, S; Ziegler, M; Buhner, M; et al. Psychiatrists' use of shared decision making in the treatment of schizophrenia: patient characteristics and decision topics. *Psychiatric services* (Washington, DC)., 2009, 60(8), 1107-12.

[47] Benbassat, J; Pilpel, D; Tidhar, M. Patients' preferences for participation in clinical decision making: a review of published surveys. *Behavioral medicine* (Washington, DC)., 1998, 24(2), 81-8.

[48] Patel, SR; Bakken, S; Ruland, C. Recent advances in shared decision making for mental health. *Current opinion in psychiatry.*, 2008, 21(6), 606-12.

[49] Goossensen, A; Zijlstra, P; Koopmanschap, M. Measuring shared decision making processes in psychiatry: skills versus patient satisfaction. *Patient education and counseling.*, 2007, 67(1-2), 50-6.

[50] Hamera, E; Pallikkathayil, L; Baker, D; White, D. Descriptive study of shared decision making about lifestyle modifications with individuals

who have psychiatric disabilities. *Journal of the American Psychiatric Nurses Association.*, 2010, 16(5), 280-7.

[51] Stewart, DC; Anthony, GB; Chesson, R. 'It's not my job. I'm the patient not the doctor': patient perspectives on medicines management in the treatment of schizophrenia. *Patient education and counseling.*, 2010, 78(2), 212-7.

[52] Young, HN; Bell, RA; Epstein, RM; Feldman, MD; Kravitz, RL. Physicians' shared decision-making behaviors in depression care. *Archives of internal medicine.*, 2008, 168(13), 1404-8.

[53] Loh, A; Simon, D; Hennig, K; Hennig, B; Harter, M; Elwyn, G. The assessment of depressive patients' involvement in decision making in audio-taped primary care consultations. *Patient education and counseling.*, 2006, 63(3), 314-8.

[54] Eisenthal, S; Emery, R; Lazare, A; Udin, H. "Adherence" and the negotiated approach to patienthood. *Archives of general psychiatry.*, 1979, 36(4), 393-8.

[55] Kent, S; Yellowlees, P. Psychiatric and social reasons for frequent rehospitalization. *Hospital & community psychiatry.*, 1994, 45(4), 347-50.

[56] Nageotte, C; Sullivan, G; Duan, N; Camp, PL. Medication compliance among the seriously mentally ill in a public mental health system. *Social psychiatry and psychiatric epidemiology.*, 1997, 32(2), 49-56.

[57] Sullivan, G; Wells, KB; Morgenstern, H; Leake, B. Identifying modifiable risk factors for rehospitalization: a case-control study of seriously mentally ill persons in Mississippi. *The American journal of psychiatry.*, 1995, 152(12), 1749-56.

[58] Fenton, WS; Blyler, CR; Heinssen, RK. Determinants of medication compliance in schizophrenia: empirical and clinical findings. *Schizophrenia bulletin.*, 1997, 23(4), 637-51.

[59] Elixhauser, A; Eisen, SA; Romeis, JC; Homan, SM. The effects of monitoring and feedback on compliance. *Medical care.*, 1990, 28(10), 882-93.

[60] Deegan, PE. The importance of personal medicine: a qualitative study of resilience in people with psychiatric disabilities. *Scandinavian journal of public health Supplement.*, 2005, 66, 29-35.

[61] Rogers, A; Day, JC; Williams, B; Randall, F; Wood, P; Healy, D; et al. The meaning and management of neuroleptic medication: a study of patients with a diagnosis of schizophrenia. *Soc Sci Med.*, 1998, 47(9), 1313-23.

[62] Cabassa, LJ; Hansen, MC; Palinkas, LA; Ell, K. Azucar y nervios: explanatory models and treatment experiences of Hispanics with diabetes and depression. *Soc Sci Med.*, 2008, 66(12), 2413-24.

[63] Usher, K. Taking neuroleptic medications as the treatment for schizophrenia: A phenomenological study. *The Australian and New Zealand journal of mental health nursing.*, 2001, 10(3), 145-55.

[64] Lieberman, JA; Stroup, TS; McEvoy, JP; Swartz, MS; Rosenheck, RA; Perkins, DO; et al. Effectiveness of antipsychotic drugs in patients with chronic schizophrenia. *The New England journal of medicine.*, 2005, 353(12), 1209-23.

[65] Deegan, PE. Recovery: The lived experience of rehabilitation. *Psychosocial Rehabilitation Journal.*, 1988, 11(4), 11-9.

[66] Klein, ERJ; Rosenber, S. Whose treament is it anyway? *The role of consumer preferences in mental health care.*, 2007.

[67] Calsyn, RJ; Winter, JP; Morse, GA. Do consumers who have a choice of treatment have better outcomes? *Community mental health journal.*, 2000, 36(2), 149-60.

[68] Cooper, J. Reducing fears and increasing assertiveness: The role of dissonance reduction. *Journal of Experimental Social Psychology.*, 1980, 16(3), 199-213.

[69] Sterling, RC; Gottheil, E; Glassman, SD; Weinstein, SP; Serota, RD. Patient treatment choice and compliance. Data from a substance abuse treatment program. *The American journal on addictions/American Academy of Psychiatrists in Alcoholism and Addictions.*, 1997, 6(2), 168-76.

[70] Joosten, EA; de Jong, CA; de Weert-van Oene, GH; Sensky, T; van der Staak, CP. Shared decision-making reduces drug use and psychiatric severity in substance-dependent patients. *Psychotherapy and psychosomatics.*, 2009, 78(4), 245-53.

[71] Bedi, N; Chilvers, C; Churchill, R; Dewey, M; Duggan, C; Fielding, K; et al. Assessing effectiveness of treatment of depression in primary care. Partially randomised preference trial. *The British journal of psychiatry; the journal of mental science.*, 2000, 177, 312-8.

[72] Silverstein, SM; Bellack, AS. A scientific agenda for the concept of recovery as it applies to schizophrenia. *Clinical psychology review.*, 2008, 28(7), 1108-24.

[73] Corrigan, PW; Faber, D; Rashid, F; Leary, M. The construct validity of empowerment among consumers of mental health services. *Schizophrenia research.*, 1999, 38(1), 77-84.

[74] McCabe, R; Priebe, S. The therapeutic relationship in the treatment of severe mental illness: a review of methods and findings. *The International journal of social psychiatry.*, 2004, 50(2), 115-28.

[75] Frank, AF; Gunderson, JG. The role of the therapeutic alliance in the treatment of schizophrenia. *Relationship to course and outcome. Archives of general psychiatry.*, 1990, 47(3), 228-36.

[76] Wong, JG; Clare, CH; Holland, AJ; Watson, PC; Gunn, M. The capacity of people with a 'mental disability' to make a health care decision. *Psychological medicine.*, 2000, 30(2), 295-306.

[77] Cortes, DE; Mulvaney-Day, N; Fortuna, L; Reinfeld, S; Alegria, M. Patient--provider communication, understanding the role of patient activation for Latinos in mental health treatment. *Health education & behavior: the official publication of the Society for Public Health Education.*, 2009, 36(1), 138-54.

[78] Nicaise, P; Lorant, V; Dubois, V. Psychiatric Advance Directives as a complex and multistage intervention, a realist systematic review. *Health & social care in the community.*, 2013, 21(1), 1-14.

[79] Campbell, LA; Kisely, SR. Advance treatment directives for people with severe mental illness. *The Cochrane database of systematic reviews.*, 2009(1), Cd005963.

[80] van Grieken, RA; Beune, EJ; Kirkenier, AC; Koeter, MW; van Zwieten, MC; Schene, AH. Patients perspectives on how treatment can impede their recovery from depression. *Journal of affective disorders.*, 2014, 167, 153-9.

[81] Stacey, D; Menard, P; Gaboury, I; Jacobsen, M; Sharif, F; Ritchie, L; et al. Decision-making needs of patients with depression: a descriptive study. *Journal of psychiatric and mental health nursing.*, 2008, 15(4), 287-95.

[82] Malpass, A; Shaw, A; Sharp, D; Walter, F; Feder, G; Ridd, M; et al. "Medication career" or "moral career"? The two sides of managing antidepressants: a meta-ethnography of patients' experience of antidepressants. *Soc Sci Med.*, 2009, 68(1), 154-68.

[83] Simmons, MB; Hetrick, SE; Jorm, AF. Experiences of treatment decision making for young people diagnosed with depressive disorders: a qualitative study in primary care and specialist mental health settings. *BMC psychiatry.*, 2011, 11(1), 1-13.

[84] Simon, D; Loh, A; Wills, CE; Harter, M. Depressed patients' perceptions of depression treatment decision-making. *Health Expect.*, 2007, 10(1), 62-74.

[85] Goldney, RD; Fisher, LJ; Wilson, DH. Mental health literacy: an impediment to the optimum treatment of major depression in the community. *Journal of affective disorders*., 2001, 64(2-3), 277-84.

[86] Dwight-Johnson, M; Unutzer, J; Sherbourne, C; Tang, L; Wells, KB. Can quality improvement programs for depression in primary care address patient preferences for treatment? *Medical care*., 2001, 39(9), 934-44.

[87] Loh, A; Kremer, N; Giersdorf, N; Jahn, H; Hanselmann, S; Bermejo, I; et al. [Information and participation interests of patients with depression in clinical decision making in primary care]. *Zeitschrift fur arztliche Fortbildung und Qualitatssicherung*., 2004, 98(2), 101-7.

[88] Raue, PJ; Schulberg, HC; Lewis-Fernandez, R; Boutin-Foster, C; Hoffman, AS; Bruce ML. Shared decision-making in the primary care treatment of late-life major depression: a needed new intervention? *International journal of geriatric psychiatry*., 2010, 25(11), 1101-11.

[89] Khalsa, SR; McCarthy, KS; Sharpless, BA; Barrett, MS; Barber, JP. Beliefs about the causes of depression and treatment preferences. *Journal of clinical psychology*., 2011, 67(6), 539-49.

[90] King, M; Sibbald, B; Ward, E; Bower, P; Lloyd, M; Gabbay, M; et al. Randomised controlled trial of non-directive counselling, cognitive-behaviour therapy and usual general practitioner care in the management of depression as well as mixed anxiety and depression in primary care. *Health technology assessment* (Winchester, England)., 2000, 4(19), 1-83.

[91] Wittink, MN; Cary, M; Tenhave, T; Baron, J; Gallo, JJ. Towards Patient-Centered Care for Depression: Conjoint Methods to Tailor Treatment Based on Preferences. *The patient*., 2010, 3(3), 145-57.

[92] Gum, AM; Arean, PA; Hunkeler, E; Tang, L; Katon, W; Hitchcock, P; et al. Depression treatment preferences in older primary care patients. *The Gerontologist*., 2006, 46(1), 14-22.

[93] Churchill, R; Khaira, M; Gretton, V; Chilvers, C; Dewey, M; Duggan, C; et al. Treating depression in general practice: factors affecting patients' treatment preferences. *The British Journal of General Practice*., 2000, 50(460), 905-6.

[94] Dwight-Johnson, M; Sherbourne, CD; Liao, D; Wells, KB. Treatment Preferences Among Depressed Primary Care Patients. *Journal of general internal medicine*., 2000, 15(8), 527-34.

[95] Jaycox, LH; Asarnow, JR; Sherbourne, CD; Rea, MM; LaBorde, AP; Wells, KB. Adolescent primary care patients' preferences for depression treatment. *Adm Policy Ment Health.*, 2006, 33(2), 198-207.

[96] Givens, JL; Houston, TK; Van Voorhees, BW; Ford, DE; Cooper, LA. Ethnicity and preferences for depression treatment. *General hospital psychiatry.*, 2007, 29(3), 182-91.

[97] Unutzer, J; Katon, W; Callahan, CM; Williams, JW; Jr. Hunkeler, E; Harpole, L; et al. Collaborative care management of late-life depression in the primary care setting: a randomized controlled trial. *Jama.*, 2002, 288(22), 2836-45.

[98] Eisenman, DP; Meredith, LS; Rhodes, H; Green, BL; Kaltman, S; Cassells, A; et al. PTSD in Latino patients: illness beliefs, treatment preferences; and implications for care. *Journal of general internal medicine.*, 2008, 23(9), 1386-92.

[99] Raue, PJ; Schulberg, HC; Heo, M; Klimstra, S; Bruce, ML. Patients' depression treatment preferences and initiation, adherence, and outcome: a randomized primary care study. *Psychiatric services* (Washington, DC)., 2009, 60(3), 337-43.

[100] Riedel-Heller, SG; Matschinger, H; Angermeyer, MC. Mental disorders--who and what might help? Help-seeking and treatment preferences of the lay public. *Social psychiatry and psychiatric epidemiology.*, 2005, 40(2), 167-74.

[101] Houle, J; Villaggi, B; Beaulieu, MD; Lesperance, F; Rondeau, G; Lambert, J. Treatment preferences in patients with first episode depression. *Journal of affective disorders.*, 2013, 147(1-3), 94-100.

[102] Lowe, B; Schulz, U; Grafe, K; Wilke, S. Medical patients' attitudes toward emotional problems and their treatment. What do they really want? *Journal of general internal medicine.*, 2006, 21(1), 39-45.

[103] Mergl, R; Henkel, V; Allgaier, AK; Kramer, D; Hautzinger, M; Kohnen, R; et al. Are treatment preferences relevant in response to serotonergic antidepressants and cognitive-behavioral therapy in depressed primary care patients? Results from a randomized controlled trial including a patients' choice arm. *Psychotherapy and psychosomatics.*, 2011, 80(1), 39-47.

[104] Cabassa, LJ; Lester, R; Zayas, LH. "It's like being in a labyrinth:" Hispanic immigrants' perceptions of depression and attitudes toward treatments. *Journal of immigrant and minority health/Center for Minority Public Health.*, 2007, 9(1), 1-16.

[105] Angermeyer, MC; Breier, P; Dietrich, S; Kenzine, D; Matschinger, H. Public attitudes toward psychiatric treatment. An international comparison. *Social psychiatry and psychiatric epidemiology.*, 2005, 40(11), 855-64.

[106] Chilvers, C; Dewey, M; Fielding, K; Gretton, V; Miller, P; Palmer, B; et al. Antidepressant drugs and generic counselling for treatment of major depression in primary care: randomised trial with patient preference arms. *BMJ: British Medical Journal.*, 2001, 322(7289), 772-5.

[107] Schneider, A; Korner, T; Mehring, M; Wensing, M; Elwyn, G; Szecsenyi, J. Impact of age, health locus of control and psychological co-morbidity on patients' preferences for shared decision making in general practice. *Patient education and counseling.*, 2006, 61(2), 292-8.

[108] Akincigil, A; Bowblis, JR; Levin, C; Walkup, JT; Jan, S; Crystal, S. Adherence to antidepressant treatment among privately insured patients diagnosed with depression. *Medical care.*, 2007, 45(4), 363-9.

[109] Sheehan, DV; Keene, MS; Eaddy, M; Krulewicz, S; Kraus, JE; Carpenter, DJ. Differences in medication adherence and healthcare resource utilization patterns: older versus newer antidepressant agents in patients with depression and/or anxiety disorders. *CNS drugs.*, 2008, 22(11), 963-73.

[110] Demyttenaere, K; Enzlin, P; Dewe, W; Boulanger, B; De Bie, J; De Troyer, W; et al. Compliance with antidepressants in a primary care setting, 1: Beyond lack of efficacy and adverse events. *The Journal of clinical psychiatry.*, 2001, 62 Suppl 22, 30-3.

[111] Pekarik, MWG. A Meta-Analysis of Psychotherapy Dropout. *Professional Psychology: Research and Practice.*, 1993, 24(2), 190-5.

[112] Gartlehner, G; Hansen, RA; Morgan, LC; Thaler, K; Lux, L; Van Noord, M; et al. Second-generation antidepressants in the pharmacologic treatment of adult depression: an update of the 2007 comparative effectiveness review [internet]. 2011.

[113] Cipriani, A; Furukawa, TA; Salanti, G; Geddes, JR; Higgins, JP; Churchill, R; et al. Comparative efficacy and acceptability of 12 new-generation antidepressants: a multiple-treatments meta-analysis. *The Lancet.*, 2009, 373(9665), 746-58.

[114] Timbie, JW; Fox, DS; Van Busum, K; Schneider, EC. Five reasons that many comparative effectiveness studies fail to change patient care and clinical practice. *Health affairs (Project Hope).*, 2012, 31(10), 2168-75.

[115] Davies, NM; Gunnell, D; Thomas, KH; Metcalfe, C; Windmeijer, F; Martin, RM. Physicians' prescribing preferences were a potential

instrument for patients' actual prescriptions of antidepressants. *J Clin Epidemiol.*, 2013, 66(12), 1386-96.

[116] Gaissmaier, W; Anderson, BL; Schulkin, J. How do physicians provide statistical information about antidepressants to hypothetical patients? *Medical decision making: an international journal of the Society for Medical Decision Making.*, 2014, 34(2), 206-15.

[117] LeBlanc, A; Herrin, J; Williams, MD; Inselman, JW; Branda, ME; Shah, ND; et al. Shared Decision Making for Antidepressants in Primary Care: A Cluster Randomized Trial. *JAMA internal medicine.*, 2015, 175(11), 1761-70.

[118] Simmons, MB; Hetrick, SE; Jorm, AF. Making decisions about treatment for young people diagnosed with depressive disorders: a qualitative study of clinicians' experiences. *BMC psychiatry.*, 2013, 13, 335.

[119] Bultman, DC; Svarstad, BL. Effects of physician communication style on client medication beliefs and adherence with antidepressant treatment. *Patient education and counseling.*, 2000, 40(2), 173-85.

[120] Lin, EH; Von Korff, M; Katon, W; Bush, T; Simon, GE; Walker, E; et al. The role of the primary care physician in patients' adherence to antidepressant therapy. *Medical care.*, 1995, 33(1), 67-74.

[121] Aikens, JE; Nease, DE; Jr. Nau, DP; Klinkman, MS; Schwenk, TL. Adherence to maintenance-phase antidepressant medication as a function of patient beliefs about medication. *Ann Fam Med.*, 2005, 3(1), 23-30.

[122] Karasz, A. The development of valid subtypes for depression in primary care settings: a preliminary study using an explanatory model approach. *The Journal of nervous and mental disease.*, 2008, 196(4), 289-96.

[123] Alverson, HS; Drake, RE; Carpenter-Song, EA; Chu, E; Ritsema, M; Smith, B. Ethnocultural variations in mental illness discourse: some implications for building therapeutic alliances. *Psychiatric services* (Washington, DC)., 2007, 58(12), 1541-6.

[124] Hickie Am, IB; Davenport, TA; Luscombe, GM; Rong, Y; Hickie, ML; Bell, MI. The assessment of depression awareness and help-seeking behaviour: experiences with the International Depression Literacy Survey. *BMC psychiatry.*, 2007, 7(1), 1-12.

[125] Nakane, Y; Jorm, AF; Yoshioka, K; Christensen, H; Nakane, H; Griffiths, KM. Public beliefs about causes and risk factors for mental disorders: a comparison of Japan and Australia. *BMC psychiatry.*, 2005, 5, 33.

[126] Shankar, BR; Saravanan, B; Jacob, KS. Explanatory models of common mental disorders among traditional healers and their patients in rural south India. *The International journal of social psychiatry.*, 2006, 52(3), 221-33.

[127] Vega, WA; Karno, M; Alegria, M; Alvidrez, J; Bernal, G; Escamilla, M; et al. Research issues for improving treatment of U.S. Hispanics with persistent mental disorders. *Psychiatric services* (Washington, DC)., 2007, 58(3), 385-94.

[128] Guarnaccia, PJ; Lewis-Fernandez, R; Marano, MR. Toward a Puerto Rican popular nosology: nervios and ataque de nervios. *Culture, medicine and psychiatry.*, 2003, 27(3), 339-66.

[129] Reiling, DM. Boundary maintenance as a barrier to mental health help-seeking for depression among the Old Order Amish. The Journal of rural health: official journal of the American Rural Health Association and the National Rural Health Care Association., 2002, 18(3), 428-36.

[130] Schiller, PL; Levin, JS. Is there a religious factor in health care utilization? *A review. Soc Sci Med.*, 1988, 27(12), 1369-79.

[131] Conrad, MM; Pacquiao, DF. Manifestation, attribution, and coping with depression among Asian Indians from the perspectives of health care practitioners. J*ournal of transcultural nursing: official journal of the Transcultural Nursing Society/Transcultural Nursing Society.*, 2005, 16(1), 32-40.

[132] Chatters, LM; Bullard, KM; Taylor, RJ; Woodward, AT; Neighbors, HW; Jackson, JS. Religious participation and DSM-IV disorders among older African Americans: findings from the National Survey of American Life. *The American journal of geriatric psychiatry: official journal of the American Association for Geriatric Psychiatry.*, 2008, 16(12), 957-65.

[133] Kiesler, DJ; Auerbach, SM. Optimal matches of patient preferences for information, decision-making and interpersonal behavior: evidence, models and interventions. *Patient education and counseling.*, 2006, 61(3), 319-41.

[134] Radford, MH; Mann, L; Kalucy, RS. Psychiatric disturbance and decision-making. *The Australian and New Zealand journal of psychiatry.*, 1986, 20(2), 210-7.

[135] Appelbaum, PS; Grisso, T; Frank, E; O'Donnell, S; Kupfer, DJ. Competence of depressed patients for consent to research. *The American journal of psychiatry.*, 1999, 156(9), 1380-4.

[136] Sayers, SL; White, T; Zubritsky, C; Oslin, DW. Family involvement in the care of healthy medical outpatients. *Family practice.*, 2006, 23(3), 317-24.

[137] Rokke, PD; Tomhave, JA; Jocic, Z. The role of client choice and target selection in self-management therapy for depression in older adults. *Psychology and aging.*, 1999, 14(1), 155-69.

[138] Williams, JW; Jr. Gerrity, M; Holsinger, T; Dobscha, S; Gaynes, B; Dietrich, A. Systematic review of multifaceted interventions to improve depression care. *General hospital psychiatry.*, 2007, 29(2), 91-116.

[139] Swanson, KA; Bastani, R; Rubenstein, LV; Meredith, LS; Ford, DE. Effect of mental health care and shared decision making on patient satisfaction in a community sample of patients with depression. *Medical care research and review: MCRR.*, 2007, 64(4), 416-30.

[140] Loh, A; Simon, D; Wills, CE; Kriston, L; Niebling, W; Harter, M. The effects of a shared decision-making intervention in primary care of depression: a cluster-randomized controlled trial. *Patient education and counseling.*, 2007, 67(3), 324-32.

[141] Ludman, E; Katon, W; Bush, T; Rutter, C; Lin, E; Simon, G; et al. Behavioural factors associated with symptom outcomes in a primary care-based depression prevention intervention trial. *Psychological medicine.*, 2003, 33(6), 1061-70.

[142] Von Korff, M; Katon, W; Rutter, C; Ludman, E; Simon, G; Lin, E; et al. Effect on disability outcomes of a depression relapse prevention program. *Psychosomatic medicine.*, 2003, 65(6), 938-43.

[143] Halter, MJ. The stigma of seeking care and depression. *Archives of psychiatric nursing.*, 2004, 18(5), 178-84.

[144] Klap, R; Unroe, KT; Unutzer, J. Caring for mental illness in the United States: a focus on older adults. *The American journal of geriatric psychiatry: official journal of the American Association for Geriatric Psychiatry.*, 2003, 11(5), 517-24.

[145] Thompson, TL; 2nd, Mitchell, WD; House, RM. Geriatric psychiatry patients' care by primary care physicians. *Psychosomatics.*, 1989, 30(1), 65-72.

[146] Unutzer, J; Katon, W; Sullivan, M; Miranda, J. Treating depressed older adults in primary care: narrowing the gap between efficacy and effectiveness. *The Milbank quarterly.*, 1999, 77(2), 225-56; 174.

INDEX

A

B

C

D

E

F

G

H

I

J

L

M

N

O

P

T

U

V